A TO Z DISEASES INFORMATION

AUTHORS
VEMPATI RAYAPAREDDY
KANURI MANIDEEPIKA

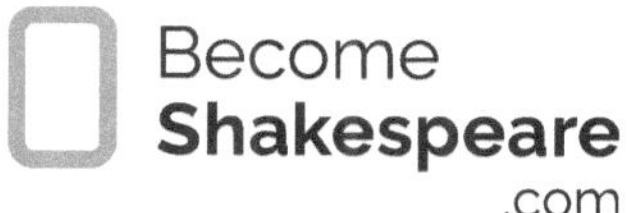

First Published in 2020

Becomeshakespeare.com

One Point Six Technologies Pvt Ltd
123, Building J2, Shram Seva Premises,
Wadala Truck Depot, Wadala (East),
Mumbai 400037, India
T: +91 8080226699

Wordit Art Fund helps deserving authors publish their work by providing monetary support. To apply for funding, please visit us at www.BecomeShakespeare.com

ISBN - 978-93-90463-36-7

PREFACE

This book contains information regarding all the diseases, from letter A to letter Z [covers 297 diseases]. The information includes Definition, Epidemiology, Pathophysiology, Risk factors, Symptoms, Diagnosis, and Treatment.

This book provides the method of easy learning to the medical and pharma students. It can also be used as reference book before attending the competitive exams and interviews.

ABOUT THE AUTHORS

VEMPATI RAYAPAREDDY

Vempati Rayapareddy is pursuing his Doctor Of Pharmacy at St. Peter's Institute of Pharmaceutical Sciences. He published 6 articles in 3 international journals [IJISRT, JETIR and IJRAR] at a very young age. He is a young, dynamic, enthusiastic and brilliant student. From his childhood, he stood as a topper in all his academics. This is a portal to introduce himself to the whole world with divine's blessings.

KANURI MANIDEEPIKA

Kanuri Manideepika is pursuing her Doctor Of Pharmacy at St. Peter's Institute of Pharmaceutical Sciences. She is a bright student from her primary education. She secured 98% in her secondary education and 97.5% in her higher education. She secured gold medal in her Pharm.D third year. She published 6 articles in 3 international journals [IJISRT, IJRAR, JETIR] at a very young age. This is a portal to introduce herself to the whole world with the divine's blessings.

CONTENTS

Letter B

Letter C

Letter D

Letter E

Contents

Letter F

Letter G

Letter H

Letter I

Letter J

Letter K

Letter L

Letter M

Contents

Letter Q

Letter R

Contents

Letter V

Letter W

Letter X

Letter Y

Letter Z

AORTIC ANEURYSM

Definition: A Aortic Aneurysm is an enlargement [dilatation] of the aorta to greater than 1.5 times normal size. They usually cause no symptoms except when ruptured. Occasionally, there may be abdominal, back or leg pain.

Epidemiology: Aortic Aneurysms resulted in about 1,52,000 deaths in 2013.

Pathophysiology: An Aortic Aneurysm can occur as a result of trauma, infection, or most commonly, from an intrinsic abnormality in the elastin and collagen components of aortic wall. While definite genetic abnormalities were identified in true genetic syndromes associated with aortic aneurysms, both thoracic and abdominal aortic aneurysms demonstrate a strong genetic component in their aetiology.

Risk Factors:
Hypertension
Tobacco use
Alcohol use
Pregnancy

Symptoms:

Most aortic aneurysms do not produce symptoms.

As they enlarge, symptoms such as abdominal pain and back pain may develop.

Compression of nerve roots may cause leg pain or numbness

Rarely, clotted blood which lines most aortic aneurysms can break off and result in embolus.

Diagnosis:

Physical examination

Medical imaging

Treatment:

Surgery [open or endovascular]

Control blood pressure using beta blockers and occasionally statins.

Small aneurysm in elderly patient with severe cardiovascular disease would not be repaired.

Endovascular treatment of aortic aneurysms is a minimally invasive alternative to open surgery repair. It involves placement of endo-vascular stent through small incisions at the top of each leg.

Open surgery starts with exposure of dilated portion of aorta via incision in the abdomen and chest followed by insertion of a synthetic graft to replace the diseased aorta.

Life Style Modifications:

Reduce the amount of sodium and cholesterol in your diet.

Eat lean meats, lots of fruits and vegetables, and wholegrains.

Avoid strenuous activities.

ACANTHAMOEBA INFECTION

Definition: Acanthamoeba keratitis is a rare but serious infection of the eye that can result in permanent visual impairment or blindness. This infection is caused by a microscopic, free-living amoeba called Acanthamoeba.

Epidemiology: The estimated rate of acanthamoeba keratitis is 1 per 2,50,000 people.

Pathophysiology:

Acanthamoeba have been found in soil, sea water, swimming pools, contact lens equipments, dental treatment units, dialysis machines. It has 2 stages, one is cysts and the other is tropozoites.

This undergoes mitosis and enters human in various ways

(1) Through the eye and causes keratitis.

(2) Through ulcerated or broken skin and cause lesions.

(3) Through nasal passage and cause lower respiratory tract infections.

(4) Sometimes reaches to central nervous system and cause granulomatous amebic encephalitis with immunocompromised individuals and infects the brain and spinal cord.

Risk factors:

Storing and handling lenses improperly

Disinfecting lenses improperly

Coming into contact with contaminated water

Having a history of trauma to the cornea.

Symptoms:

Eye pain

Eye redness

Blurred vision

Sensitivity to light

Excessive tearing

Fever

Diagnosis:

Confocal microscopy

Granulomatous amebic encephalitis is diagnosed by brain scan, biopsies or spinal tap.

Treatment:

Skin infections that are not spread to CNS can be successfully treated with combination of chlorohexidine[0.02%] and polyhexamethyl biguanide [0.02%]

Topical Miconazole

Metronidazole

Prednisolone

Neomycin

Oral ketoconazole

Life style modifications:

Reduce exposure to light

Eat Vitamin-A rich foods

Drink plenty of water.

ADENOVIRUS INFECTION

Definition: One of the group of viruses that can cause infections of the lung, stomach, intestine, and eyes.

Epidemiology: Adenovirus is a very common infection, estimated to be responsible for 2% to 5% of all respiratory infections.

Pathophysiology: Adenoviruses infect and replicate in the epithelial cells of the: pharynx, conjunctiva, urinary bladder, small intestine.

They usually donot spread beyond the regional lymph nodes except in the immune compromised host.

Adenoviruses cause infections in: respiratory tract, eye, urinary bladder and intestine.

Risk factors:

History of chronic disease

History of recent transplantation

Immunocompromised

Symptoms:

Common cold

Sore throat

Bronchitis

Pneumonia

Diarrhoea

Pink eye

Fever

Diagnosis:

Antigen detection, Polymerase chain reaction assay, virus isolation and serology.

Treatment:

Antivirals

Ribavirin

Cidofovir

Ganciclovir

Vidarabine

ACQUIRED IMMUNO DEFICIENCY SYNDROME [AIDS]

Definition: Fatal illness caused by a retrovirus HIV. It breaks down the body's immune system, leaving the potential vulnerable to a host of life threatening opportunistic infections, neurological disorders or unusual malignancies.

Epidemiology:

Males>females

Occurs in all ages and ethnic groups

All areas of the country are affected.

Pathophysiology:

Binding to CD4 internalization and internalization which leads to uncoating and reverse transcriptase and integrated proviral DNA which causes productive infection, mature HIV production and cell lysis.

Risk factors:

Unprotected sex

Contaminated needles and syringes

Symptoms:

Follow this pattern:

Acute illness

Asymptomatic period

Advanced infection

Diagnosis:

HIV antibody test

Viral antigen test

Detection of viral nucleic acid in blood

Determining the CD4 counts.

Treatment:

NRTI:

Zidovudine

Lamivudine

Stavudine

Didanosine

Zalcitabine

Abacavir

Tenofivir

Emtricitabine

NNRTI:

Nevirapine

Efavirenz

Delavirdine

Integrase inhibitors

Raltegravir

PI:

Indinavir

Nelfinavir

Saquinavir

Ritonavir

Life style modifications:

Avoid multiple partners

Use sterile needles each time for infection

Never share needles

Avoid unnecessary blood transfusions.

All pregnant women should be tested for HIV.

ATTENTION DEFICIT HYPERACTIVITY DISORDER

Definition: ADHD is a problem with inactiveness, over activity, impulsivity or a combination.

Epidemiology: ADHD affects people of all ages.

Pathophysiology: The neurotransmitters dopamine and norepinephrine are complicated in the pathophysiology of ADHD. Dopamine is a neurotransmitter involved in reward, risk taking, impulsivity and mood. Norepinephrine modulates attention, arousal and mood.

Risk factors:

Exposure to environmental toxins- such as lead, found mainly in paint and pipes in older building.

Maternal drug use

Alcohol use and smoking

Symptoms:

ADHD symptoms generally improve with age. However, adults who were diagnosed at an early age may continue to experience some symptoms and their associated problems. To be diagnosed with ADHD, your child will have atleast 6 symptoms of inactiveness.

Diagnosis:

There is no single test to diagnose ADHD. It can be diagnosed after a person has shown some or all of the symptoms of ADHD on a regular basis for more than 6 months.

Treatment:

There are 5 types of medication licensed for treatment of ADHD:

Methylphenidate

Dexamfetamine

Lis dexamfetamine

Atomoxetine

Guanfacine

Parent education and training programmes:

They can help you learn ways to speak, work and play with your child to improve their behavior and attention span.

ATRIAL FIBRILLATION

Definition: Atrial fibrillation, is an irregular, rapid heartbeat that may cause symptoms like heart palpitations, fatigue and shortness of breath.

Epidemiology:

The incidence of AF ranges between 0.21 and 0.41 per 1000 per year. Permanent AF occurs approximately 50% of patients, paroxysmal and persistent AF in 25% each. AF is frequently associated with cardiac diseases and co-morbidities.

Pathophysiology:

The prevalence of AF, already the most common sustained cardiac arrhythmia, is constantly rising, even after adjusting for age and presence of structural heart disease.

Risk factors:

High blood pressure

Valvular heart disease

Coronary artery disease

Cardiomyopathy

Congenital heart disease
COPD
Smoking
Sleep apnea

Symptoms:

Unpleasant palpitations or irregularity of heart beat
Mild chest discomfort
A sense of heart racing
Light headedness
Difficult breathing
Shortness of breath
Confusion

Diagnosis:

Feeling the pulse
Electrocardiogram

Treatment :

Beta blockers : slows heart rate, decreases blood pressure

Calcium channel blockers: relaxes blood vessels

Antiarrhythmic agents: helps control abnormal heart rhythms

Blood thinners: helps prevent blood clots from forming or helps dissolve existing clots.

AFRICAN TRYPANOSOMIASIS

Definition:

It is also called as African sleeping disease or sleeping sickness. It is transmitted by bite of tse-tse fly.

Epidemiology:

It is a chronic form of disease present in western and central Africa.

Pathophysiology:

It is caused by 2 subspecies of the flagella protozoan Trypanosoma brucei, which are transmitted to human hosts by bites of infected tse-tse flies.

Risk factors:

Ingestion of contaminated water

Receiving blood transfusions

Receiving organ donation from individuals.

Symptoms:

Pain areas

Insomnia

Weight loss

Fever

Headache

Itching

Mental confusion

Skin rash

Diagnosis:

Finding the parasite in body fluid or tissue by microscopy.

Treatment :

The current treatment for T.b.gambiense is IV or IM Pentamidine.

The treatment for T.b rhodesiense is IV suramin

Patient counselling:

Closely monitoring the neurological condition.

Control of airway may be required to prevent aspiration.

Monitoring of hepatic and renal function.

ALKHURMA HAEMORRHAGIC FEVER

Definition:

AHF is caused by alkhurma haemorrhagic fever virus, a tick borne virus of flavivirus family.

Epidemiology:

Contact with domestic animals or livestock may increase the risk of human infections.

No human to human transmission has been documented.

Pathophysiology:

Although livestock animals may provide blood meals for ticks, it is tough that they play minor role in transmitting AHFV to humans. No transmission through non-pasteurized milk has been described, although other tick borne flaviviruses have been transmitted to humans through this route.

Risk factors:

Contact with livestock with tick exposure

Slaughtering of animals

Symptoms:

Fever

Anorexia

General malaise

Diarrhoea

Vomiting

Neurological and hemorrhagic symptoms in severe case

Diagnosis:

Molecular detection by PCR

Serological test using ELISA.

Treatment:

No standard specific treatment for the disease

Patients receive supportive therapy, which consists of balancing the fluids and electrolytes

Maintaining oxygen status and blood pressure.

Patient counselling:

Individuals should use tick repellants on skin and clothes.

People working with animals or animal products should avoid unprotected contact with blood, fluids, or tissues of any potentially infected or viremic animals.

AMYOTROPIC LATERAL SCLEROSIS

Definition:

It is a group of rare neurological diseases that mainly involve the nerve cells responsible for controlling voluntary muscle movement. Motor neurons are nerve cells that extent from the brain to spinal cord and to muscles throughout the body.

Epidemiology:

It is seen in higher age groups.

Pathophysiology:

ALS is the most common degenerative disease of motor neuron system. The disorder is named for its underlying pathophysiology, with amyotrophy referring to atrophy of muscle fibers, which are denervated as their corresponding anterior horn cells degenerate.

Risk factors:

Heredity

Age[40-60]

Sex[men]

Genetics

Symptoms:

Difficulty in walking

Tripping and falling

Weakness in your legs, feet and ankles.

Hand weakness

Slurred speech

Muscle cramps

Diagnosis;

Electromyogram [EGM]

Spinal tap

Muscle biopsy

Magnetic resonance imaging [MRI]

Blood and urine tests

Nerve conduction study

Treatment:

Riluzole – slows the disease progression in some people, by reducing levels of chemical messenger in the brain.

Edaravone – given via IV infusion.

ALZHEIMER'S DISEASE

Definition:

Alzheimer's disease is an irreversible, progressive brain disease that slowly destroys memory and disorders cognitive function.

Epidemiology:

Morethan 25 million people in the world today are affected by dementia, most suffering from alzheimers disease.

Pathophysiology:

Due to etiological factors, changes that occur in proteins of nervecells of cerebral cortex which leads to accumulation of neurofibrillary tangles and plaques that leads to granulovascular degeneration and loss of cholinergic nerve cells and finally loss of memory, function and cognition.

Risk factors:

Down's syndrome
Chronic high BP
Family history

Head injuries

Smoking and drinking

Symptoms:

Confusion

Personality changes

Language difficulties

Disturbances in short term memory

Unexplained mood swings

Diagnosis:

CT scan

MRI

PET

SPECT

ECG

CSF examination

Mental status examination

Psychiatric assessments

Treatment:

Acetyl cholinesterase inhibitors

Anti depressants

Anxiolytics

Antipsychotics

Anti convulsants

Patient counselling:

Crisis intervention counselling

Individual counselling

Family therapy

Group therapy

Long term residential treatment

Self help

AMOEBIASIS

Definition:

Amoebiasis is a disease caused by one celled parasite called Entamoeba histolytica

Epidemiology:

Amoebiasis is estimated to cause 70,000 deaths per year

Pathophysiology:

Amoebiasis is transmitted by fecal contamination of drinking water and foods but also by direct contact with dirty hands or objects as well as by sexual contact.

Risk factors:

Stress

Alcoholism

Malnutrition

Immunodeficiency

Alternation of bacterial flora

Corticosteroid therapy

Symptoms:

Abscesses

Infection

Severe illness

Death

Diagnosis:

Indirect haemagglutination assay [IHA]

ELISA

Latex agglutination test

Gel diffusion

Counter current immunoelectrophoresis

Treatment:

Treatment for uncomplicated cases of amebiasis generally consists of 10-day course of metronidazole that you take as a capsule.

Surgery may be necessary if the colon or peritoneal tissues have perforations.

Patient counselling:

Thoroughly wash fruits and vegetables before eating.

Avoid ice cubes.

Avoid milk, cheese or other unpasteurized dairy products.

Avoid food sold by street vendors.

AMERICAN TRYPANOSOMIASIS

Definition:

Chagas disease is an inflammatory, infectious disease caused by parasite Trypanosoma cruzi, which is found in the feces, it is also called as American trypanosomiasis.

Epidemiology:

It can infect anyone.

It is found in south America and the south and south western USA.

Pathophysiology:

The pathophysiology process is characterized by inflammatory response, cellular lesions and then fibrosis. It affects the heart, oesophagus, and colon most severely. The cardiomyopathy that it shows high levels of fibrosis. An inflammatory process is autonomic denervation. In the heart, conducting system is also destroyed.

Risk factors:

80% of transmission is by insect vector

5-20% transmission is by blood transfusion or transplantation.

Symptoms:

Fever

Flu like symptoms

Rash

Swollen eye lid

Diagnosis:

ECG

Chest X ray

Echocardiogram

Abdominal X ray

Upper endoscopy

Treatment:

Treatment with anti parasitic drugs benznidazole and nifurtimox kills or inhibits T.Cruzi parasites.

Chronic phase patients are usually treated using treatments directed at specific symptoms or organ damage.

Patient counselling:

Bedrest is adviced at severe acute phase

Stop alcohol consumption.

ANAPLASMOSIS

Definition: It is a disease caused by rickettsial parasite of ruminants. The micro organism is gram negative, and infect red bloodcells.

Epidemiology :

It can infect anyone

Pathophysiology:

Clinical bovine anaplasmosis is caused by A marginale. Cattle are also infected with A centrale, which generally results in mild disease. A ovis may cause mild to severe disease in sheep, dear and goats.

Risk factors:

People become infected by eating undercooked or contaminated meat.

Symptoms:

Fever

Severe headaches

Muscle aches

Chills and shaking

Less frequent symptoms include nausea, vomiting, weightloss and loss of appetite.

Diagnosis:

PCR

Treatment:

Doxycycline

Use of antibiotics other than doxycycline or tetracycline have been associated with higher risk of fatal outcome.

Patient counselling:

Eat hygienic food.

ANCYCLOSTOMA DUODENATE INFECTION

Definition:

Ancyclostoma infection: hookworm, an intestinal parasite that usually causes diarrhea and cramps. Hook worms have a complex life cycle that begins and ends in the small intestine. Hook worm eggs require warm, moist, shaded soil to hatch into larvae.

Epidemiology:

Distribution is world wide but mostly in areas with a moist, warm climate.

Pathophysiology:

This is a GI infection characterized by chronic blood loss that leads to iron deficiency anaemia and protein malnutrition. It is caused primarily by N americanus and A duodenate and less commonly by zoonotic species A ceylonium.

Risk factors:

Poor personal hygiene, particularly defecation particles and sanitation have been reported as risk factors of hookworm infection.

Symptoms:

Itchiness

Localized rash

Abdominal pain

Diarrhea

Diagnosis:

Stool sample

Treatment:

Albendazole

Mebendazole

Improve nutrition

Treat complications from anemia

Patient counselling:

Iron supplementation

Proper hygienic conditions.

ANISAKIS INFECTION

Definition: It is a genus of parasitic nematodes, which have a cycle involving fish and marine animals. They are infective to humans and cause anisakiasis.

Epidemiology:

Mostly seen in fishing areas

Increasing incidence in North America

Pathophysiology:

It affects human by the process of ingestion of seal fish and cephalopods. It have a life cycle involving fish and marine animals.

Risk factors:

Fishing areas and fish size are risk factors of anisakis infection.

Symptoms:

GI symptoms

Allergy-type reactions

Diagnosis:

Direct visualization

Removal of larvae via gastroscopy

Serological testing

Imaging studies

Treatment:

Infection that can lead to small bowel obstruction, which may require surgery, although there are case reports of treatment with albendazole alone being successful. Intestinal perforation is also possible.

ANTHRAX

Definition: It is a serious infectious disease caused by gram-positive, rod shaped bacteria knoen as Bacillus anthracis.

Epidemiology:

Soil is contaminated with anthrax spores from carcasses of dead animals.

Pathophysiology :

It may cause infections in the regions of skin, inhalational and gastrointestinal.

Risk factors:

Environmental exposure

Occupational exposure

Biologic terrorism

Undercooked meat ingestion

Heroin use

Symptoms:

Symptoms of anthrax depends on the type of infection.

Diagnosis:

Gram staining

Test of infected skin

Blood testing

CT scans

Chest X ray

Endoscopy of intestine

Treatment :

Many antibiotics are effective against anthrax in humans, but treatment must be started early.

Ciprofloxacin is recommended for treatment.

Pencillin G, along with gentamicin or streptomycin, has previously used to treat anthrax.

ARENA VIRUS

Definition:

The infection which is caused by Arena virus, is a virus which is a member of the family Arenaviridae.

Epidemiology:

The arenavirus that affect humans exist in natue as benign infections in restricted rodent hosts.

Pathophysiology:

Chronic infection in rodent host

Human infection occurs by contact with rodent excretions

Secondary spread [person-person]

Zoonotic

Risk factors:

Age

Race

Symptoms:

Pyrexia

Headache

Sore throat

Myalgia

Diagnosis:

Virus isolation

Virus neutralization

Detection of antibodies

PCR technology

Treatment:

Ribavirin [anti-viral]

The sooner treatment is started after infection, the better the chances of survival.

Patient counselling:

Avoid contact with rodents.

ARTHRITIS

Definition:

A disease causing painful inflammation and stiffness to the joints.

Epidemiology:

The prevalence of arthritis is relatively constant in many populations.

Pathophysiology:

In arthritis, the body's immune system attacks the lining of the joint capsule, a tough membrane that encloses all the joint parts. This lining becomes inflamed and swollen. The disease process can eventually destroy cartilage and bone within the joint.

Risk factors:

Non-modifiable: age, gender, heredity

Modifiable: obesity, diabetes

Symptoms:

Fatigue

Joint pain

Joint stiffness

Diagnosis:

Diagnose your arthritis by asking you about your symptoms and how they have developed, examining you and possibly arranging for tests to be done.

C-reactive protein

ESR

Treatment:

Analgesics

NSAID'S

Counter irritants

Biologic response modifier

Corticosteroids

Patient counselling:

Weight loss

Exercise

Heat and cold

Assistive devices

ASCARIS INFECTION

Definition:

Infection that is caused by ascaris. It is the most common helminthic human infection.

Epidemiology:

Indiscriminate defecation particularly near areas of habitation seeds the soil with eggs.

Pathophysiology:

Migration of larvae

Little damage is caused by the penetration

Some larvae migrate to ectopic sites and dependent upon number and location, cause various inflammatory responses, leading to very severe allergic reactions.

Transplacental migration can also occur

Risk factors:

It is found in association with poor personal hygiene, poor sanitation, and where human feces are used as fertilizer.

Symptoms:

Coughing

Wheezing

Aspiration pneumonia

Blood in mucus

Chest discomfort

Fever

Diagnosis:

Macroscopic identification

Larval worms

Stool microscopy

Ultrasound

Treatment:

Albendazole: a single oral dose of 400mg

Mebendazole: 100mg orally twice daily for 3 days

Piperazine

Pyrantel pamoate

Ivermectin

ANAEMIA

Definition: A condition in which the blood doesn't have enough healthy red blood cells.

Epidemiology:

More than 10 million cases per year[in india]

Pathophysiology:

Anemia caused by blood loss

Caused by decreased or faulty blood cell production

Bone marrow and stem cells problems.

Types:

Iron deficiency anemia

Sickle cell anemia

Vitamin deficiency anemia

Anemia associated with other chronic conditions

Hemolytic anemia

Pernicious anemia

Risk factors:

Lack of vitamins and minerals

Family history

Symptoms:

Dizziness

Light headedness

Unusual heart beat

Cold hands and feet

Tiredness or weakness

Diagnosis:

Haemoglobin

Complete blood picture

Complete blood count

Treatment:

Folic acid supplements

Iron supplements

Bone marrow transplant in severe cases.

ASTHMA

Definition:

A disease characterized by an increased responsiveness of the airways to various stimuli resulting in airway obstruction that is reversible either spontaneous or as a result of treatment.

Epidemiology:

By 1 year: 26%

1 to 5 years: 51.4%

Morethan 5 years: 22.3%

Pathophysiology:

Asthma is a common pulmonary condition defined by chronic inflammation of respiratory tubes, tightening of respiratory smooth muscles, and episodes of bronchoconstriction.

Risk factors:

Sensitization to allergen

Maternal diet during pregnancy and lactation

Pollutants

Microbes and their products

Psychosocial factors

Symptoms:

Cough : 90%

Wheezing : 74%

Exercise induced wheeze or cough : 55%

Diagnosis:

General attitude and well being

Deformity of the chest

Character of breathing

Thorough ausculatation of breath sounds

Treatment:

Controllers are medications to be taken on daily long term basis.

Relievers are medications to be used on needed basis to relieve symptoms quickly

Bronchodilators are mostly used to treat asthma.

Life style modifications:

Avoid strenuous exercises

Avoid citrus foods

Avoid eating chocolates, ice creams, and spicy foods.

AUTISM

Definition:

It is defined by the presence of abnormal or impaired development that is manifested before the age of 3 years characterized by abnormalities of social development, communication and a restriction of behavior and interest.

Epidemiology:

Typically appears during the first 3 years of life.

Pathophysiology:

Autism spectrum disorder [ASD] manifests in early childhood and is characterized by qualitative abnormalities in social interactions.

Risk factors:

Myotoxins

c-sections

maternal antibodies

placental abnormalities

smoking

air pollution

endocrine disrupters

Symptoms:

Poor eye contact

Impairment in visual tracking to an object

Atypical responsiveness to name

Less social smiling

Delayed expressive and receptive language

Diagnosis:

Presently, we don't have a medical test that can diagnose autism. Instead, specially trained physicians and psychologists administer autism-specific behavioural evaluations.

Treatment:

Therapy includes a wide range of tools, services and teaching methods.

AVIAN INFLUENZA

Definition: It is also called as bird-flu. These viruses occur naturally among wild aquatic birds.

Epidemiology:

Avian influenza is a slightly misleading term, as influenza is among the natural infections found in birds.

Pathophysiology:

Pathology of H5N1 avian influenza is responsible for bird flu.

Risk factors:

Poultry farmer

A traveler visiting affected areas

Exposed to infected birds

Someone who eats undercooked poultry or eggs

Symptoms:

Cough

Diarrhea

Respiratory difficulties

Fever

Headache

Muscle aches

Malaise

Runny nose

Diagnosis:

Rapid diagnostic tests for identifying avian influenza A[H7N9] virus in clinical samples.

Treatment:

Tamiflu, an antiviral drug, appears to be effective in treating bird flu.

ASEPTIC MENINGITIS

Definition: It is the inflammation of the meninges, a membrane covering the brain and spinal cord in patients whose cerebro spinal fluid tests negative with routine bacterial cultures. The most common cause of aseptic meningitis is by viral infection.

Epidemiology:

The incidence of aseptic meningitis has been reported as 11 per 1lakh persons a year.

Pathophysiology:

The mechanisms by which circulating viruses penetrate the blood brain barrier and cause inflammatory response, but to a lesser degree than bacterial infection does.

Risk factors:

Viruses

Fungi

Tuberculosis

Worms

Some medications

Infections near the brain and spinal cord

Symptoms:

Pain in the areas like back, muscles, neck.

Fever

Chills

Loss of appetite

Nausea

Vomiting

Skin rashes

Irritability

Headache

Mental confusion

Diagnosis:

Blood cultures

CT scans to check for brain swelling

Chest X ray

Treatment:

Most people with aseptic meningitis recover in one to two weeks without medical treatment.

Analgesics and anti-inflammatory medications may be recommended for pain and fever control.

Patient counselling:

A life style that includes a balanced diet, adequate sleep, appropriate exercise and the avoidance of excessive stress is very important.

Avoid inhalation of cigarette smoke.

B VIRUS INFECTION [HERPES B VIRUS]

Definition:

B virus infection is caused by a herpes virus B. virus. Macaque monkeys are thought to be the natural host for the virus.

Epidemiology:

The study found no evidence of B.virus infection among 130 close contacts of 4 patients, health care workers.

Pathophysiology:

Primary infection of B virus in primates is similar to herpes simplex virus1 infection in human beings, but B virus generally produce only mild localized lesions in the natural host. In human beings, however, B virus can cause severe infection that may lead to death from encephalitis.

Risk factors:

Occupational exposure

Travel to countries with free-roaming macaques

Keeping macaques as pets

Exposure to non-macaque species that have been housed with macaques.

Symptoms:

Vesicular skin lesions

Localized neurological symptoms

Flu like aches

Fever

Chills

Fatigue

Diagnosis:

Serology

PCR

Brain CT

CSF tests

Brain MRI

Treatment:

Ganciclovir

Acyclovir

Patient counselling:

The ability of therapy to prevent herpes B virus infection is not documented, and therapy can suppress shedding and seroconversion, further complicating diagnosis.

BURKHOLDERIA CEPACIA INFECTION

Definition:

Burkholderia cepacia is an aerobic gram-negative bacillus found in various aquatic environments.

Epidemiology:

Preliminary studies indicate that certain of these species are more likely to colonize and cause severe pulmonary infection in person with cystic fibrosis.

Pathophysiology:

Burkholderia cepacia is a pathogen usually causing infection to immune-compromised or hospitalized patients. It is also associated with infections in patients with underlying lung disease, such as cystic fibrosis and chronic granulomatous disease.

Risk factors:

Chronic lung infections are the most prevalent cause of premature death in patients with C.F.

Symptoms:

Increased cough
Congestion

Fever

Difficulty breathing

Diagnosis:

Detoriation of lung tissue

X ray

Treatment:

Carbapenems

Ceftazidime

Chloramphenicol

Fluoroquinolones

Piperacillin

Trimethoprim- sulfamethoxazole.

BABESIA INFECTION

Definition:

Babesiosis is a malaria-like parasitic disease caused by infection with bacteria.

Epidemiology:

The epidemiology of babesiosis in general depended on several parameters such as availability of host, presence of ticks that act as vector for transmission of infections.

Pathophysiology:

Infected erythrocytes eventually rupture and release merozoites invade other erythrocytes. The main pathogenesis associated with babesiosis is hemolytic anemia. Hemolytic anemia is a result of direct erythrocyte injury caused by the parasites and also by immune-mediated mechanisms.

Risk factors:

Increasing age

Concurrent lyme disease

Immunosuppression

Symptoms:

Fatigue

Severe headache

Muscle aches

Joint pain

Abdominal pain

Nausea

Diagnosis:

Giesma – stained thin-film blood smear

Treatment:

Babesia is a parasite and wont respond to antibiotics alone.

Treatment requires anti parasitic drugs, such as those used for malaria.

Atovaquone plus azithromycin is used to treat most cases and is usually taken for 7-10 days.

Clindamycin plus quinine is used in more severe cases.

Patient counselling:

Wear clothing treated with permethrin

Wear long pants and long sleeved shirts.

BACTERIAL MENINGITIS

Definition:

Meningitis is an inflammation of the membranes [meninges] surrounding the brain and spinal cord.

Epidemiology:

Over 1.2 million cases of bacterial meningitis are estimated to occur worldwide each year.

Pathophysiology:

The organisms usually enter the meninges through the blood stream from other parts of the body. Bacterial meningitis consists of pyogenic inflammation of the meninges and the underlying subarachnoid CSF.

Risk factors:

Alcoholism

Auto immune disorders

Conditions like HIV, AIDS

Immunosuppressive drugs

Intravenous drug abuse

Removal of spleen

Smoking

Symptoms:

Pain areas: back, muscle, neck

Fever

Chills

Lethargy

Loss of appetite

Malaise

Nausea

Vomiting

Red rashes

Diagnosis:

Blood cultures

Imaging [CT,MRI]

Spinal tap

Treatment:

Age: 0-4weeks: ampicillin + cefotaxime or aminoglycosides

Age: 1 month – 50 years: vanomycin + cefotaxime or ceftriaxone

Age: above 50 years: vancomycin + ampicillin+ ceftriaxone or cefotaxime.

BACTERIAL VAGINOSIS

Definition:

Bacterial vaginosis [BV] is a disease of vagina caused by excessive growth of bacteria.

Epidemiology:

Prevalence of BV increases based on lifetime member of sexual partners.

Pathophysiology:

The normally predominant lactobacilli population is reduced in vagina, while populations of Gardnerella vaginalis and other anaerobes are increased.

Risk factors:

Having multiple sex partners or a new sex partner

Douching

Natural lack of lactobacilli bacteria

Symptoms:

Thin, gray, white or green vaginal discharge

Foul smelling 'fishy' vaginal odour

Vaginal itching

Burning during urination

Diagnosis:

Gram's stain

Cytology

Culture

Commercial tests

PCR based assays

Whiff test

Treatment:

Metronidazole

Clindamycin

Tinidazole

Patient counselling:

Advice avoidance of vaginal douching

Advice against the use of shower gel.

BALAMUTHIA INFECTION

Definition:

Balamuthia infection is a cutaneous condition resulting from balamuthia that may result in various skin lesions.

Epidemiology:

Balamuthia species has been found in the soil and water. Infection probably occurs from inhalation of contaminated water or soil.

Pathophysiology:

Balamuthia causes a slow, insidious, and chronic diseases like that caused by Acanthamoeba and may develop over a period of time from about 2 weeks to 2 years. Infections with balamuthia have occurred in immunocompromised hosts, including HIV, AIDS patients and immunocompetent individuals.

Risk factors:

HIV, AIDS

Cancer

Liver disease

Diabetes mellitus

Symptoms:

Head ache

Stiff neck

Sensitivity to light

Nausea

Vomiting

Lethargy

Low grade fever

Diagnosis:

Immune fluorescence assay [IFA]

Immuno histochemistry [IHC]

Treatment:

Flucytosine

Pentamidine

Fluconazole

Sulfadiazine

Azithromycin or clarithromycin.

BALANTIDIUM INFECTION

Definition:

Balantidium coli is an intestinal protozoan parasite that causes the infection.

Epidemiology:

Almost all of the children surveyed were infection with one or more parasites in addition to Balantidium coli

Pathophysiology:

Balantidium coli is an intestinal protozoan parasite that causes the infection. While this type of infection is uncommon in U.S, humans and other mammals can become infected with Balantidium coli by ingesting infective cysts from food and water that is contaminated by feces.

Risk factors:

Close contact with pigs

Tropical and subtropical regions

Poor hygiene

Crowded or institutional living conditions

Zookeeper.

Symptoms:

Mostly asymptomatic

Balantidium infection can cause symptoms as diarrhea and abdominal pain.

Diagnosis:

Stool examination

Treatment:

Tetracycline
Metronidazole
Iodoquinol.

BARTONELLA BACILLIFORMIS INFECTION

Definition:

Bartonella bacilliformis is a highly infectious agent causing sandfly- disseminated disease, oroya fever and verruga peruana in parts of south America.

Epidemiology:

The incidence of infection was 12.7/100persons/year.

Pathophysiology:

Both B henselae and B.quintana may cause bacillary angiomatosis, infections in homeless populations and infections in patients with HIV.

Risk factors:

Flea infestation

Symptoms:

Fever

Headache

Rash

Bone pain

Diagnosis:

Thin blood smear

Treatment:

The combination of doxycycline and rifampin is preferred for the treatment of patients.

ARTONELLA QUINTANA INFECTION

Definition:

This micro organism is transmitted by human body louse and is causative agent of well known tench fever

Epidemiology:

Homeless populations

Infections in patients with HIV

Pathophysiology:

Both B.hensekea, and B.quintana may cause bacillary angiomatosis infections in homeless populations and infections in patients with HIV.

Risk factors:

Poor living conditions
Chronic alcoholism

Symptoms:

Fever

Fatigue

Headache

Loss of appetite

Rash

Swollen glands

Diagnosis:

Blood smear

Treatment:

Doxycycline orally for 6 weeks in combination with gentamycin in intravenous daily dose for 14 days.

BAYLISASCARIS INFECTION

Definition:

This infection is caused by raccoon round worm

Epidemiology:

Raccoons become infected with Baylisascaaris in one of the 2 ways: adult raccoons acquire the infection by eeating rodents, rabbits and birds infected with larvae of Baylisascaris

Pathophysiology:

It is the most common cause of clinical larva migrans in animals, in which it is usually associated with fatal or severe neurological disease.

Risk factors:

Young children

Symptoms:

Nausea

Tiredness

Liver enlargement

Loss of co ordination

Lack of attention to people and surroundings

Lack of muscle control

Blindness

Coma

Diagnosis:

Eye examinations may reveal a migrating larva or lesions

Treatment:

Albendazole [20-40mg/kg/day for 1-4weeks] has been used to treat many cases.

BILHARZIA

Definition:

A chronic disease, endemic in parts of Africa and south ameica caused by infestation with blood flukes [schistosomes]

Epidemiology:

Globally 2,00,000 deaths are attributed to schistosomiasis annually.

Pathophysiology:

When larval forms of parasites, released by freshwater snails, penetrate their skin during contact with infested water. In the body, the larvae develop into adult schistosomes. Adult worms live in blood vessels, where the female release eggs.

Risk factors:

Poor sanitation

Symptoms:

abdominal, joint and muscle pain

Pain may occur during sexual intercourse

Blood in stools

Diarrhea

Chills

Fatigue

Fever

Frequent urination

Blood in urine

Cough

Headache

Diagnosis:

Stool or urine samples can be examined microscopically for parasitic eggs.

Treatment:

Amoscanate

Arteether

Artemether

Chloroxylenol

Hycanthone

Lucanthone

Meclonazepam

Corticosteroids.

BLASTOCYSTIS INFECTION

Definition:

This infection in stools of people who have diarrhea, abdominal pain or other gastrointestinal problems.

Epidemiology:

Seen in children who live in crowded settings

Pathophysiology:

Certain forms may be more likely to an infection. It is also found in stools of people who have diarrhea, abdominal pain or gastrointestinal problems.

Risk factors:

Increased age, height, weight

HIV

Symptoms:

Diarrhea

Nausea

Abdominal cramps

Bloating

Excessive gas

Loss of appetite

Fatigue

Diagnosis:

Microscopic examination of stool samples

Treatment:

Metronidazole

Tinidazole

Combination medication such as sulfamethoxazole and trimethoprim.

Patient counselling:

Wash hands thoroughly using soap.

Avoid food or water

Wash and peel all raw vegetables and fruits before eating.

BORRELIA BURGDOFERI INFECTION

Definition:

Lyme disease is caused by Borrelia burgdoferi and is transmitted to humans through the bite of infected black legged ticks.

Epidemiology:

Primarily in united states

Pathophysiology:

Certain investigators suggest that transmission of the spirochetes occur via infectious saliva, although in light of fact that only 5% of adult ticks are systemically infected,.

Risk factors:

Who spend time in grassy and heavily wooded areas

Symptoms:

Fever

Headache

Fatigue

Characteristic skin rash

Diagnosis:

Serological tests do not become positive until an infected individual has had time to develop antibodies.

Treatment:

Doxycycline

Amoxicillin

Cefuroxime axetil.

BOTULISM

Definition:

Food poisoning caused by bacterium growing on improperly sterilized thinned meats and other preserved foods.

Epidemiology:

Current understanding of the epidemiology of a botulism outbreak relies on limited data from very few reports.

Pathophysiology:

Wound botulism results from contamination of wound with toxin producing C botulism.

Risk factors:

Who eat low-canned low acidic foods

Drug users

Symptoms:

Abdominal pain

Constipation

Nausea

Vomiting

Dilated pupil

Fatigue

Mouth dryness

Blurred vision

Difficulty speaking

Diagnosis:

Analysis of blood, stool, or vomit for evidence of toxin

Treatment:

Guanethidine and 4-aminopyridine

Local antibiotics such as pencillin G or metronidazole.

BOVINE SPONGIFORM ENCEPHALOPATHY

Definition:

Also called mad cow disease

A brain disorder in adult cattle that may be spread to humans through diseased meat.

Epidemiology:

Fewer than 5000 cases per year

Pathophysiology:

Convincing evidence indicates that variant creulzfeldt-jakob disease is a new disease. Despite its name, variant CSD appears to be a human variant of BSE derived from a cow-to-human species switch, rather than actual variant of human sporadic CJD.

Risk factors:

People who consume contaminated beef

Symptoms:

Depression

Dementia

Loss of co-ordination

Diagnosis:

MRI

Treatment:

Trimipramine – antidepressant

Fluphenazine – antipsychotic.

BRAINERD DIARRHEA

Definition:

It is a syndrome of acute onset of watery diarrhea lasting for 4 weeks or longer which can occur in outbreaks or as sporadic cases.

Epidemiology:

All age groups

Pathophysiology:

Brainerd diarrhea is a syndrome of acute onset of watery diarrhea. Patient typically experience 10-20 episodes per day of explosive , watery diarrhea characterized by urgency and often by fecal incontinence.

Risk factors:

Contaminated food and water

Symptoms:

Watery non bloody diarrhea with urgency

Fetal incontinence

Gas

Mild abdominal cramping

Fatigue

Diagnosis:

Examining the patient condition

Treatment:

Anti microbic agents

Anti inflammatory agents.

BREAST CANCER

Definition:

Breast cancer starts when cells in the breast begin to grow out of control.

Epidemiology:

1,82,000 women diagnosed with breast cancer annually.

Pathophysiology:

Breast cancer refers to several types of neoplasm arising from breast tissue.

Risk factors:

Women

Increased age

Genetics

Symptoms:

May not cause any symptoms

A lump may be too small for you to feel

Rash

Discharge from nipple

Pain in the breast

Diagnosis:

Breast biopsy

Mammograms

Ultrasound

MRI

Treatment:

Depends on stage of your breast cancer

Chemotherapy

Hormone therapy

HER2 target drugs such as Herceptin, parjeta.

BRONCHIOLITIS

Definition:

Bronchiolitis is an acute viral infection of the small air passages of lungs called bronchioles.

Epidemiology:

About 75% of cases of bronchiolitis occur in children younger than1year and 95% in children younger than 2 years.

Pathophysiology:

Acute infection of epithelial cells lining the small airways within the lungs.

Risk factors:

Pre mature birth

Symptoms:

Fast breathing

Shortness of breath

Wheezing

Dehydration

Fever

Loss of appetite

Diagnosis:

Urine or blood tests

A small electronic device is clipped to your child's finger toe to measure the oxygen in blood.

Treatment:

Airway support

Supplemental oxygen

Support of fluids

Ribavirin

Nebulized bronchodilators

Corticosteroids

Patient counselling:

Supportive care

Adequate fluid and nutrition management.

BRONCHITIS

Definition:

Inflammation of mucus membrane in the bronchial tubes

Epidemiology:

Acute bronchitis affected 44 of 1000 adults annually

Pathophysiology:

Increased mucus production along with edema of the bronchus

Risk factor:

Cigarette smoke

Symptoms:

Cough

Fatigue

Malaise

Runny nose

Chest tightness

Headache

Shortness of breath

Diagnosis:

Stethoscope

Chest X ray

Treatment:

Plenty of rest

Drinks lot of fluids

Paracetamol

Ibuprofen.

BRUCELLA INFECTION

Definition:

Brucellosis is an infectious disease caused by a type of bacteria called brucella.

Epidemiology:

World wide

Pathophysiology:

The bacteria are transmitted from animals to humans by ingestion through infected food products, direct contact with an infected animal, or inhalation of aerosols.

Risk factors:

Occupational exposure

Unpasteurized dairy products consumption

Consumption of raw meat products

Symptoms:

Abdominal, muscle, joint, backpain
Fever

Chills

Fatigue

Loss of appetite

Loss of weight

Coughing

Headache

Swollen lymphnodes

Diagnosis:

Blood tests

Treatment:

Aminoglycoside therapy in conjunction with doxycycline, rifampin and TMP-SMZ for atleast 4weeks, followed by atleast 2-3 active agents without aminoglycosides for another 8-12 weeks is preferred.

Chronic brucellosis is treated with triple antibiotic therapy.

BURKHOLDERIA PSEUDOMALLEI INFECTION

Definition:

Melioidosis is an infectious disease caused by gram-negative bacterium, Burkholderia pseudomallei

Epidemiology:

B.pseudomallei is present in soil and water and cause infection

Pathophysiology:

It is spread to humans through direct contact with a contaminated source, especially during the rainy season.

Risk factors:

Diabetes

Excessive alcohol use

Chronic renal disease

Chronic lung disease

Thalassemia

Non-HIV related immunosupressent

Symptoms:

Chest pain and joint pain

Cough

Skin infections

Lung nodules

Pneumonia

Diagnosis:

Diagnosed with the help of blood, urine, sputum, skin
–lesion testing.

Treatment:

Intensive phase:

Parenteral ceftazidime, amoxicillin-clavulanic acid

Eradication phase:

Oral trimethoprim- sulfamethoxazole.

CLOSTRIDIUM DIFFICILE INFECTION

Definition:

Most common causes of infection of colon

Epidemiology:

Worldwide

Pathophysiology:

Disturbance of normal bacterial flora of the colon release toxins and cause mucosal inflammation and damage.

Risk factors:

Increasing age

Non surgical gastro intestinal diseases

Symptoms:

Abdominal pain

Diarrhea

Bloating

Blood in stools

Fever

Diagnosis:

Stool test

Treatment:

Antibiotic

Metronidazole-orally.

CAMPYLOBACTER INFECTION

Definition:

Most common bacterial infection of human

Epidemiology:

Worldwide

Pathophysiology:

Infection can lead to extraintestinal disease and severe long term complications.

Risk factors:

Food specific

Consumption of chicken prepared at a commercial food establishment.

Symptoms:

Diarrhea

Fever

Nausea

Vomiting

Abdominal pain

Headache

Muscle pain

Diagnosis:

Test detects:

Stool test

Body tissue or fluids

Treatment:

IV

Erythromycin.

CANCER

Definition;

A disease caused by an uncontrolled division of abnormal cells in a part of the body.

Epidemiology:

Cancer epidemiology is dedicated to increasing understanding about cancer causes, prevention and control.

Pathophysiology:

Carcinogenesis:

Cancers are caused by series of mutations.

Risk factors:

Family history

Diet

Alcohol

Tobacco use

Exposure to sunlight, radiation

Symptoms:

Fatigue

Weight changes

Lump or area of thickening

Skin changes

Diagnosis:

Physical exam

Laboratory tests

Imaging tests: CT, MRI, PET, ultrasound, Xray

Biopsy

Treatment:

Surgery

Chemotherapy

Radiation therapy

Stem cell production

Immunotherapy

Hormone therapy

Targeted drug therapy

Clinical trials.

CANDIDA INFECTION

Definition:

Candidiasis is a fungal infection due to any type of candida.

Epidemiology:

The increase in infections due to candida over the past decade is significant.

Pathophysiology:

Candida infections of the skin and superficial mucosal sites are the result of an interplay between fungal virulence and host defenses.

Risk factors:

Immunosuppression

Diabetes

Corticosteroids

Symptoms:

White patches or vaginal discharge

Itchy

Diagnosis:

Yeast infections are simple to diagnose.

Treatment:

Clotrimazole

Nystatin

Fluconazole.

CANINE FLU

Definition:

Canine influenza [dog flu] is influenza occurring in canine animals.

Epidemiology:

An overview of the epidemiology and emergence of influenza A infection in humans overtime.

Pathophysiology:

Canine influenza viruses causes an acute respiratory infection in dogs

Risk factors:

Exposure to influenza virus

Symptoms:

Upper respiratory illness

Runny nose

Congestion

Malaise

Diagnosis:

PCR performed on deep nasal or pharyngeal swabs

Treatment:

Currently, there is an approved vaccine in the US for canine influenza, but it is only for the AH3N8 strain of the virus. At this time, there is no vaccine available for the H3N2 canine flu virus.

CAPILLARIA INFECTION

Definition:

Capillariasis is a parasitic infection caused by 2 species of nematodes.

Epidemiology:

Most cases have been recognized in the Philippines, where the infection was first noted in 1960.

Pathophysiology:

Capillaria philippinensis causes a malabsorption enteropathy that may be severe and even fatal.

Risk factors:

Risk behaviours

Associated conditions

Protective factors

Symptoms:

Sneezing and nasal discharge

Coughing

Wheezing

Painful urination and incontinence

Diagnosis:

The specific diagnosis of capillaria philippinensis infection requires the demonstration of c

Treatment:

Albendazole 400mg once daily for 10 days

Mebendazole 200mg once daily for 20 days.

CARBAPENEM RESISTANT KLEBSIELLA PNEUMONIA

Definition:

Increased incidence of multidrug resistant gram negative infection has resulted in high rates of morbidity and mortality.

Epidemiology:

It has become a wide spread concern

Pathophysiology:

It is a gram negative infection

Risk factors:

CR-KP colonization is important to prevent spread.

Symptoms:

Pneumonia

Blood stream infections

Wound infections

Surgical site infections

Meningitis

UTI

Diagnosis:

Carbapenemase detection

Phenotypic tests

PCR

DNA micro assays

Treatment:

Aminoglycosides

Polymyxins

Tigecycline

Fosfomycin

Temocillin.

CARBAPENEM RESISTANT ENTERO BACTERIACEAE

Definition:

CRE are bacteria that have developed resistance to multiple antibiotics, including carbapenem.

Epidemiology:

Over the past 10 years, it has lead to an increase in the prevalence of CRE in the united states.

Pathophysiology:

CRE bacteria develop when genetic material develops resistant mechanisms to antibiotics and is then transferred to other bacteria.

Risk factors:

Contact with a person infected with CRE

Symptoms:

UTI

Cyanosis

Sepsis

Pneumonia

Fever

Septic shock

Low blood pressure

Diagnosis:

PCR

Treatment:

It is difficult and should involve a consult with an infectious disease specialist to help determine what mix of antibiotics may be the best choice for each individual.

CARPAL TUNNEL SYNDROME

Definition:

CTS is a collection of symptoms and signs that occurs following entrapment of the median nerve within the carpal tunnel.

Epidemiology:

Race: whites are at high risk

Sex: female:male [10:1]

Age:45-60 years

Pathophysiology:

The tendons of the hands are wrapped with a lining that produce a synovial fluid which lubricates the tendons with repetitive movement of hand, lubrication system may malfunction. This reduction in lubrication results in inflammation and swelling of tendon area. Abnormally high carpal tunnel pressures exist in patient's with CTS.

Risk factors:

Genetics

Diabetes

Thyroid

Symptoms:

Obstruction to venous outflow

Back pressure

Edema formation

Ischemia in the nerve

Diagnosis:

Physical examination

Nerve conduction studies

Treatment:

NSAID'S

Vitamin B supplements

Steroid injection.

CCHF [Crimean-congo hemorrhagic fever]

Definition:

CCHF is a wide spread tick-borne viral disease.

Epidemiology:

Primary host: zoonotic disease carried by several domestic and wild animals

Transmission: by hyalomma tick

Human: infected by tick bite

Pathophysiology:

Transmission to humans occur through contact with infected ticks or animal blood.

Risk factors:

Tick bite

Symptoms:

Swollen and painful liver

Acute kidney failure

Acute respiratory distress syndrome

Diagnosis:

ELISA

RT-PCR

Viral isolation attempts

Treatment:

Supportive therapy

Ribavirin.

CERVICAL DERMATITIS

Definition:

An itchy inflammation caused by infestation of the skin by cercariae

Epidemiology:

Prevalence in north

Pathophysiology:

After penetration of the cercaria

'Swimmers itch' if cercaria from birds involved

Risk factors:

Swimmers

Symptoms:

Tingling, burning, or itching on your exposed skin

Small, red pimples

Blisters

Diagnosis:

Physical examination

No specific tests

Treatment:

Anti-itch lotion or corticosteroid cream

Cool compress

Baths with baking soda.

CEREBRAL PALSY

Definition:

A condition marked by impaired muscle co ordination and disabilities, typically caused by damage to the brain before or at birth.

Epidemiology:

Population based studies from around the world report prevalence estimates of CP ranging from 1.5 to more than 4 per 1000 live births or children of a defined age range.

Pathophysiology:

Non progressive disorders of movement and posture, the most common cause of severe neurodisability in children. Understanding the pathophysiology is crucial to developing some protective stratergies.

Risk factors:

Brain injury or brain malformation

Symptoms:

Difficulty in bodily movements

Learning disability

Speech disorders

Constipation

Hearing loss

Leaking of urine

Diagnosis:

CT scan

MRI

EEG

Treatment:

Baclofen

Diazepam

Botox.

CERVICAL CANCER

Definition:

Cervical cancer is a type of cancer that occurs in the cervix.

Epidemiology:

12000 new cases were being diagnosed every year.

Pathophysiology:

Abnormal growth of cells that have the ability to invade or spread to other parts of the body.

Risk factors:

HPV infection

Immune system deficiency

Herpes

Smoking

Age

Socio economic factors

Symptoms:

Pain in the pelvis

Pain during sexual intercourse

Abnormal menstruation

Abnormal vaginal bleeding

Fatigue

Weight loss

Diagnosis:

PAP Test

HPV DNA test

Treatment:

Chemodrugs:

Cisplatin

Carboplatin

Paclitaxel

Topotecan

Gemcitabine.

CHAGAS DISEASE

This is also known as American trypanosomiasis

Refer disease number 12

CHAPARE HEMORRHAGIV FEVER

Definition:

CCHF is caused by chapare virus, a single stranded RNA virus of the Arenaviridae family.

Epidemiology:

A single fatal case yielded the only clinical description and blood spectrum to date

Pathophysiology:

CCHF comes from a small, poorly described cluster of hemorrhagic fever cases in rural Bolivia.

Risk factors:

Exposure to virus

Symptoms:

Fever

Headache

Articulation

Muscle pain

Vomiting

Diagnosis:

CCHF virus has been successfully isolated from both blood and serum during the acute febrile phase of illness

Treatment:

Ribavirin.

CHICKEN POX

Definition:

An infectious disease causing a mild fever and a rash of inflamed pimples which turn to blisters and then loose scabs.

Epidemiology:

The epidemiology of varicella has changed dramatically since the introduction of varicella vaccine in 1995

Pathophysiology:

After initial inhalation of contaminated respiratory droplets, the virus infects the conjunctivae or the mucosa of the upper respiratory tractr

Risk factors:

Haven't been vaccinated for chicken pox

Symptoms:

Fever

Loss of appetite

Headache

Tiredness

Diagnosis:

Self diagnosable

The most characteristic syndrome is an itchy, blister like rash on the skin

Treatment:

Acyclovir [antiviral drug].

CHICKENGUNYA FEVER

Definition:

A viral disease resembling dengue, transmitted by mosquitoes

Epidemiology:

Transmitted to humans primarily via the bite of an infected mosquito

Pathophysiology:

The infection has a clinical presentation that overlaps with that of the Ross River virus infection and dengue fever virus transmitted by the same mosquitoes.

Risk factors:

Age more than 58 years

Exposure to mosquitoes

Symptoms:

Abdominal pain

Joint pain

Muscle pain

Fever

Chills

Fatigue

Headache

Skin rash

Diagnosis:

Testing serum or plasma to detect virus

Treatment:

There is no vaccine to prevent or medicine to treat

Treat the symptoms:

Get plenty of rest

Drink fluids

Take medicine such as acetaminophen

Donot take aspirin, NSAID'S.

CHLAMYDIA TRACHOMATIS DISEASE

Definition:

It is sexually transmitted infection caused by the bacterium Chlamydia trachomatis

Epidemiology:

Sexually transmitted infection mainly of gay men, in the developed world.

Pathophysiology:

It is an obligate intracellular bacterium with a gram negative cellwall. It generally infects the columnar epithelium cells of urethra and often becomes chronic, lasting months to morethan a year, if untreated. The lifecycle of C.trachomatis is approximately 48-72 hours

Risk factors:

HIV

AIDS

PID

Symptoms:

Pain in the eyes, lower abdomen, pelvis

Pain during intercourse

Abnormal vaginal discharge

Eye discharge

Diagnosis:

Urine test

Women: swab of your discharge

Treatment:

1g dose of azithromycin orally

Doxycycline at a dosage of 100mg orally twice per day for 7 days.

CHRONIC OBSTRUCTIVE PULMONARY DISORDER

Definition:

COPD is a type of obstructive lung disease characterized by long term breathing problems and poor airflow.

Epidemiology:

Study of COPD and its determinants at the population level., aims to quantify the burden of COPD on society and to compare it with other diseases.

Pathophysiology:

Poorly reversible airflow obstruction

Abnormal inflammatory response in the lungs

Risk factors:

Long term exposure to dust and chemicals.

Symptoms:

Cough

Shortness of breath

Wheezing

Fatigue

Chest tightness

Weight loss

Diagnosis:

Spirometry

Treatment:

Aclidinium

Arformoterol

Formoterol

Glycopyrrolate

Indacaterol

Tiotropium.

CHOLERA

Definition:

An infectious and often fatal bacterial disease of the small intestine, typically contracted from infected water supplies and causing severe vomiting and diarrhea.

Epidemiology:

Developing countries

Pathophysiology:

The disease is caused by intestinal infection, with Vibrio cholera, which is highly motile gram-negative bacterium with single-sheathed flagellum.

Risk factors:

Poor sanitary conditions

Symptoms:

Abdominal pain

Nausea

Severe diarrhea

Vomiting

Dehydration

Diagnosis:

Bacteria in stool sample

Treatment:

Anti microbial agents

Tetracycline

Doxycycline

Furazolidone

Ciprofloxacin.

CLONORCHIS INFECTION

Definition:

Clonorchis sinensis, the Chinese liver fluke, is a human liver fluke.

Epidemiology:

Over 15 million are infected worldwide.

Pathophysiology:

When larvae of C.sinensis reach the biliary system and mature, the flukes provoke pathological changes, both as a result of local trauma and of local irritation.

Risk factors:

Hepatitis B

Hepatitis C

Alcoholic liver disease

Symptoms:

Fever

Chills

Epigastric pain

Tender hepatomegaly

Diarrhea

Mild jaundice

Diagnosis:

Identifying eggs in the feces or duodenal contents

Treatment:

Albendazole

Praziquantel.

CLOSTRIDIUM BOTULISM INFECTION

Botulism is a rare but serious condition caused by toxins from bacteria called clostridium botulism.

For further information refer botulism disease [disease number 38]

CLOSTRIDIUM DIFFICILE INFECTION

Definition:

A bacterium that is one of the most common causes of infection of the colon.

Epidemiology:

In the past 10-15 years, C.difficile infection has emerged as an increasingly important infectious disease worldwide.

Pathophysiology:

Colonization with C.difficile will release toxins and cause mucosal inflammation and damage.

Risk factors:

Increasing age

Non surgical gastrointestinal procedures

Anti ulcer medications

Symptoms:

Abdominal pain

Diarrhea

Bloating

Blood in stool

Fever

Diagnosis:

Stool examination

Enzyme immunoassay

Treatment:

Metronidazole

Vancomycin.

CLOSTRIDIUM TETANI INFECTION

Definition:

Clostridium tetani is the bacteria responsible for the often fatal disease tetanus.

Epidemiology:

Clostridium tetani, the spores of which are wide spread in the environment.

Pathophysiology:

The active anaerobic bacteria lead to the production of tetanus toxin, which enters the nervous system via lower motor neurons and travels upto the spinal cord and brain stem.

Risk factors:

Everyone is susceptible

Symptoms:

Jaw cramping

Sudden involuntary muscle tightening

Painful muscle stiffness all over the body

Trouble swallowing

Seizures

Headache

Fever

Sweating

Changes in blood pressure

Fast heart rate

Diagnosis:

Primarily based on patient's clinical symptoms

Microbiological tests

Treatment:

Pencillin

Metronidazole

Erythromycin

Tetracycline

Chloramphenicol

Clindamycin.

CMV
[
CYTOMEGALOVIRUS
INFECTION]

Definition:

CMV infection is common herpes virus infection with a wide range of symptoms.

Epidemiology:

Worldwide

Pathophysiology:

The molecular mechanisms responsible for the tissue damage caused by CMV.

Risk factors:

Exposure to young children

Recent onset of sexual activity

Symptoms:

Jaundice

Pneumonia

Red spots under the skin

Rash

Enlarged liver

Enlarged spleen

Low birth weight

Seizures

Diagnosis:

New born's: urine, saliva, blood or other body tissues within 2 or 3 weeks after birth

Treatment:
Antiviral drugs:

Valganciclovir

Ganciclovir

Cidofovir.

COCCIDIOIDOMYCOSIS

Definition:

It is primarily pulmonary disease.

Epidemiology:

About 60% of the infections in the endemic area are asymptomatic.

Pathophysiology:

The inflammatory reaction is both purulent and granulomatous recently released endospores incite a polymorphonyclear response.

As the endospores mature into spherules, the acute reaction is replaced by lymphocytes, plasma cells, epithelioid cells and giant cells.

Risk factors:

Exposure to dust worms or areas where soil is being disturbed.

Symptoms:

Anorexia

Weight loss

Cough

Hemoptysis

Diagnosis:

Complement-fixation

Slide-agglutination

Immunodiffusion

Treatment:

Anti-fungal therapy.

COLORODO TICK FEVER [CTF]

Definition:

Colorodo tick fever is a viral infection transmitted through a bite from an infected dermacentor andersoni wood tick.

Epidemiology:

The disease occurs almost exclusively in the western united states and southwestern Canada

Pathophysiology:

The cause of Colorado tick fever is infection with the causative agent that is transmitted by a tick-bite. This agent is a double-stranded RNA virus of the genus coltivirus.

Risk factors:

Living or travelling in rocky mountain forest areas

Symptoms:

Fever upto 105degree Fahrenheit

Chills

Severe headache

Light sensitivity

Muscle aches

Skin tenderness

Loss of appetite

Nausea

Diagnosis:

It can have incubation period of upto 20days

Treatment:

There is no specific treatment

Symptoms are treated.

COLON CANCER

Definition:

Cancer to colon

Epidemiology:

In the US, colon cancer is the 3rd leading type of cancer in males and 4th in females.

Pathophysiology:

Abnormal growth of cells

Risk factors:

Inflammatory bowel disease

Crohn's disease

Symptoms:

Abdominal pain

Blood in stool

Constipation

Fatigue

Abdominal discomfort

Weight loss

Diagnosis:

Colonoscopy

Treatment:

Avastin

Bevacizumab

Camptosar

Cetuximab

Eloxatin.

CONCUSSION

Definition:

Temporary unconsciousness or confusion and other symptoms caused by a blow on the head.

Epidemiology:

Millions of people every year

Pathophysiology:

Induced by traumatic biomechanical forces secondary to direct or indirect forces on the head.

Risk factors:

High risk sport

Symptoms:

Head ache

Fatigue

Amnesia

Disorientation

Mild depression

Sleep disturbances

Nausea

Vomiting

Diagnosis:

MRI

Treatment:

Ibuprofen

Acetaminophen.

CONJUCTIVITIS

Definition:

Inflammation of the conjunctiva of the eye.

Epidemiology:

More common in children

Pathophysiology:

Conjunctivitis, the conjunctival tissue is infiltrated by eosinophils, neutrophils, and a small number of T cells, probably recruited as a result of release of chemokines that attract these cells to the site of inflammation during the persistent, allergen driven inflammatory response.

Risk factors:

Trees and grass

Symptoms:

Inflammation of the conjunctiva

Redness

Itching

Tearing of eyes

Diagnosis:

Self diagnosable

Treatment:

Topic antibiotic therapy.

COOLEY'S ANEMIA

Definition:

Inherited disorder of hemoglobin synthesis

Epidemiology:

1 per 1lakh worldwide

Pathophysiology:

The significant excess of free chains caused by the deficiency of beta chains causes destruction of the RBC precursors in the bone marrow.

Risk factors:

Genetic disorders

Symptoms:

Feeling tired

Pale skin

Enlarged spleen

Yellowish skin

Dark urine

Diagnosis:

Blood sample

Treatment:

Blood transfusions

Iron chelation

Folic acid.

CROHN'S DISEASE

Definition:

Crohn's disease is an idiopathic inflammatory bowel disease characterized by transmural non caseating granulomatous inflammation.

Epidemiology:

Sex: male=female

Age: onset :15-30 years, another peak: 60-70 years

Pathophysiology:

Increased permeability of mucus membrane

Antigenic stimulation in the intestinal mucosa and cause physiological inflammation and cause extensive tissue injury and finally crohn's disease.

Risk factors:

Smoking

Symptoms:

Abdominal pain

Diarrhea

Low grade fever

Acute onset resembling appendicitis

Diagnosis:

Capsule endoscopy

Colonoscopy

Radiologic studies

Treatment:

No specific treatment

Treatment is given to treat symptoms.

CRYPTOSPORIDIUM INFECTION

Definition:

Infection caused by cryptosporidium spore producing parasite found in the intestine of infected people and animals

Epidemiology:

Worldwide

Pathophysiology:

Buries into intestinal lining of the gut

Alters osmotic pressure

Atrophy of intestinal villi

Risk factors:

Ingesting food or drinks contaminated with fecal material

Symptoms:

Diarrhea

Stomach cramps

Dehydration

Nausea

Vomiting

Fever

Weightloss

Sometimes no symptoms are seen

Diagnosis:

PCR

Modified acid-fast stain

Treatment:

Nitazoxanide

Paromomycin

Azithromycin.

CHRONIC WASTING DISEASE

Definition:

It is a contagious neurological disease affecting deer, elk and moose.

Epidemiology:

Forest areas

Pathophysiology:

It is fatal, endemic prion disease of wild deer, elk and moose

Symptoms:

Behavioural changes

Loss of awareness

Increased drinking

Polyuria

Excessive salivation

Diagnosis:

Necropsy

Treatment:

2-aminothiazole.

COVID-19

Definition:

It is a disease caused by new strain of coronavirus.

Epidemiology:

Spread worldwide

Pathophysiology:

It enters the humanbeings via angiotensin receptors and infect the lungs mostly.

Risk factors:

Contact with covid 19 people

Being unhygienic

Symptoms:

Fever

Loss of smell

Loss of taste

Headache

Sore throat

Cough

Cold

Bodypains

Generalized weakness

Diagnosis:

RT-PCR

[nasal and throat swabs]

Treatment:

Remedesivir

Fabiflu

Azithromycin

Ceftum

Treat symptoms

Life style modifications:

Wear mask

Maintain physical distance

Eat vitamin-c foods

Frequent sanitization.

DEEP VEIN THROMBOSIS

Definition:

DVT is the development of thrombi in the deep veins of extremitis or pelvis.

Epidemiology:

Annual incidence in urban population is 2cases per 1000persons

Pathophysiology:

Prolonged stasis

Coagulation abnormalities

Vessel wall trauma

Risk factors:

Prolonged immobilization

Postoperative state

Trauma to pelvis

Birth control pills

Symptoms:

Leg swelling

Pain

Warmth

Diagnosis:

Ultrasonography

Venography

Serum concentrations

ESR

Treatment:

IV unfractioned heparin

Enoxaparin

Dalteparin.

DENGUE FEVER

Definition:

A debilitating viral disease of the tropics, transmitted by mosquitoes and causing sudden fever and acute pains in the joints.

Epidemiology:

DHF was first documented only in the 1950's during epidemics in the Philippines and Thailand.

Pathophysiology:

Infection with any of the DENV serotypes may be asymptomatic in majority of cases.

Risk factors:

Travelling in tropical areas

Exposure to the virus

Symptoms:

Severe abdominal pain

Vomiting

Bleeding from your gums, nose

Blood in your urine

Difficult breathing

Diagnosis:

Based on symptoms, prescribe blood tests

Complete blood picture

Treatment:

Acetaminophen

NSAID'S

Ibuprofen

Naproxen sodium.

DERMATOPHYTIC INFECTION

Definition:

Infection caused by dermatophytes, fungus that require keratin for growth.

Epidemiology:

The exception is Trichophyton tonsurans related tinea capitatis in north America.

Pathophysiology:

Caused by T.rubrum may involve beyond the stratum corneum to involve the follicles, progressing to form chronic inflammatory lesions.

Risk factors:

Xerosis

Symptoms:

Itching

Rash

Nail discolouration

Diagnosis:

Microbiological studies

Treatment:

Antifungal agents:

Azoles

Allyl amines

Nystatin – not effective.

DIABETES

Definition:

A disease in which the body's ability to produce or respond to the hormone insulin is impaired, resulting in abnormal metabolism of carbohydrates and elevated levels of glucose in blood.

Epidemiology:

Worldwide

More in men

Pathophysiology:

Reduced insulin production

Insulin resistance

Types:

Insulin dependent diabetes mellitus

Non-insulin dependent diabetes mellitus

Diabetes insipidus

Gestational diabetes

Risk factors:

Over weight

Inactivity

Family history

High bloodpressure

Symptoms:

Polyuria

Polydipsia

Polyphagia

Blurry vision

Extreme fatigue

Diagnosis:

Random blood sugar

Fasting blood sugar

Post prandial blood sugar

HBA1C

Treatment:

Type 1:

Insulin

Human mixtard

Type 2:

Sulfonyl ureases

Meglitinides

Biguanides

Thiazolidine diones.

DIENTAMOEBA FRAGILIS INFECTION

Definition:

Dientamoeba fragilis is a non flagellate trichomonad parasite and is one of the smaller parasites that can live in the human large intestine.

Epidemiology:

Worldwide

Pathophysiology:

Its lifecycle has no cyst stage, thus, infection between humans occurs during the tropozoite stage.

Risk factors:

Exposure

Symptoms:

Diarrhea

Abdominal pain

Loss of appetite

Weight loss

Nausea

Fatigue

Diagnosis:

Stool sample

Treatment:

Nitroimidazole drugs:

Metronidazole

Iodoquinol

Paromomycin

Ornidazole.

DIPHYLLOBOTHRIUM INFECTION

Definition:

Infection caused by diphyllobothrium

Epidemiology:

50 million people worldwide

Pathophysiology:

It is caused by ingestion of raw or undercooked infected fish and subsequent intestinal infection.

Risk factors:

Ingestion of raw or undercooked infected fish

Symptoms:

Mostly asymptomatic

Abdominal discomfort

Diarrhea

Vomiting

Weight loss

Vitamin B12 deficiency

Anemia

Diagnosis:

Identification of egg or segments of tapeworm in stool sample.

Treatment:

Praziquantel

Niclosamide.

DIROFILARIASIS

Definition:

Infestation with filarial worms of the genus Dirofilaria and especially with the heart worm.

Epidemiology:

Worldwide

Pathophysiology:

Appearance of pulmonary coin lesion secondary to Dirofilaria immitis infection in a man

Risk factors:

Increasing prevalence rates of dirofilaria infections in domestic and wild animals.

Symptoms:

Cough

Chestpain

Fever

Pleural effusion

Diagnosis:

Open lung biopsy

Treatment:

Tetracyclines

Doxycycline

Ivermectin.

DOG BITE

Definition:

The main medical issues to be addressed with dogbites are the skin damage, only injury to underlying tissue and the significant potential for infection of the wound.

Epidemiology:

25 persons per 1000population

Pathophysiology:

The better the vascular supply and the easier the wound is to clean, the lower the risk of the infection.

Risk factors:

Areas where dogs are prevalent

Symptoms:

Bleeding

Bruising

Infection

Redness

Swelling

Pus or fluid oozing from the wound

Diagnosis:

Physical examination

Treatment:

Tetanus

Rabies prophylaxis.

DOWN SYNDROME

Definition:

A congenital disorder arising from a chromosome defect, causing intellectual impairment and physical abnormalities including short stature and broad facial profile.

Epidemiology:

One in every 1000 births

Pathophysiology:

Trisomy of chromosome 21

Risk factor:

Genetics

Symptoms:

Delayed development

Intellectual impairment

Physical impairment

Diagnosis:

Chorionic villus sampling

Treatment:

No specific treatment

Treat symptoms.

DRACUNCULIASIS

Definition:

Infection caused by guinea worm

Epidemiology:

Most prominent in south sudan

Pathophysiology:

If the larvae come into contact with water as they are emerging, the female worms discharge their larvae, setting in motion a new life cycle.

Risk factors:

Exposure

Symptoms:

Diarrhea

Nausea

Vomiting

Fever

Itching

Worm emerging from a skin blister

Diagnosis:

Diagnosis is by inspection

Treatment:

Analgesics

Aspirin

Ibuprofen

Metronidazole

Thiabendazole.

E.COLI INFECTION

Definition:

Infection caused by Escherichia coli, which is a gram-negative facultative anaerobes, rod shaped bacteria,

Epidemiology:

Worldwide

Pathophysiology:

This is a strain of E.coli that produces cytotoxins that disrupt protein synthesis within hostcells.

Risk factors:

Increased age

Weekened immune system

Symptoms:

Abdominal cramping

Severe watery diarrhea

Gas

Loss of appetite

Vomiting

Fever

Fatigue

Diagnosis:

PCR

Treatment:

Homecare is all that's required to treat an E.coli infection.

EAR INFECTION

Definition:

An ear infection is an inflammation of the middle ear, usually caused by bacteria, that occurs when fluid buildsup behind the ear drum.

Epidemiology:

Children get more often

Pathophysiology:

Inflammation of middle ear, usually caused by bacteria that occurs when fluid buildup behind the eardrum.

Risk factors:

Exposure to microorganisms

Symptoms:

Acute otitis media

Otitis media with effusion

Red bulging eardrum

Diagnosis:

Pneumatic otoscope

Tympanometry

Treatment:

Amoxicillin

Acetaminophen

Ibuprofen.

EASTERN EQUINE ENCEPHALITIS [EEE]

Definition:

A mosquito-borne viral disease

Epidemiology:

Worldwide

EEE was first recognized in USA.

Pathophysiology:

Mosquito to birds is a primary transmission cycle and it spreads to human and horse.

Risk factors:

Spending time in areas where mosquitoes are present

Symptoms:

High fever

Nervous signs

Brain lesions

Photophobia

Seizures

Diagnosis:

Isolation of virus

ELISA

Treatment:

Corticosteroids

Anti convulsants

Supporting measures such as IV fluids, tracheal incubation and antipyretics.

EBOLA VIRUS DISEASE

Definition:

Ebola virus disease is a disease caused by ebola virus in severe fatality rate, 90% affects human and non human primtes.

Epidemiology:

Western areas

Pathophysiology:

Every tissues are affected, except bones and muscles

The virus creates blood clots

Clots goes towards internal organs

It prevents oxygen to rise tissues

The virus also destroys connective tissue

Risk factors:

When come into contact with:

Blood

Secretions

Organs

Other body fluids of infected animals

Symptoms:

High temperature

Muscle pain

Nausea

Abdominal pain

Loss of appetite

Rashes

Increased liver enzyme activity

Diagnosis:

ELISA

RT-PCR

Electron microscopy

Virus isolation

Treatment:

There is no specific treatment

Treat symptoms.

EHRLICHIOSIS

Definition:

Ehrlichiosis is a group of diseases usually named according to the host species and the type of white blood cell most often onfected.

Epidemiology:

Worldwide

Mostly southeast, southcentral US, japan, malasia

Pathophysiology:

Transmission via ticks

Risk factors:

Insect bites

Symptoms:

Head ache

Fever

Malaise

Gastrointestinal signs

Diagnosis:
IFA
ELISA
PCR

Treatment:
Antibiotics:
Tetracyclines
Doxycycline.

ELEPHANTIASIS

Definition:

Abnormal accumulation of watery fluid in the tissues causing severe swelling.

Epidemiology:

Endemic in 83 countries

Pathophysiology:

Abnormal accumulation of watery fluids in the tissues which cause severe swelling

Risk factors:

Living for longtime in tropical and subtropical areas

Symptoms:

Swelling of legs, genitals, breast, and arms.

Diagnosis:

Xrays

Ultrasounds

Treatment:

Anti parasitic drugs

Diethyl carbamazine

Albendazole.

ENDOPHTHALMITIS

Definition:

Endophthalmitis is defined as an intra ocular inflammation which predominantly affects the inner spaces of eye and their contents

Epidemiology:

Worldwide

Pathophysiology:

Bacterial entry into eye cause cascade of inflammatory products and release of digestive enzymes and toxins by bacteria and cause tissue destruction.

Risk factors:

Exposure to bacteria

Symptoms:

Blurred vision

Red eye

Pain

Swollen lid

Photophobia

Diagnosis:

Ocular examination

Vitreous fluid biopsy

Neuroimaging

Treatment:

Antibiotic therapy

Antifungals.

ENTAMOEBA HISTOLYTICA INFECTION

Refer amoebiasis [disease 11]

ENTEROVIRUS INFECTION

Definition:

Infection caused by enterovirus [rotavirus]

Epidemiology:

130 million episodes per year in the world

Pathophysiology:

Infects mature enterocytes and cause atrophy and compensatory repopulation by immature secretor cells and secondary hyperplasia

Risk factors:

Exposure to virus

Consuming contaminated food and water.

Symptoms:

Often no symptoms

Sore throat

Vomiting

Fever

Diagnosis:

PCR

Treatment:

Unfortunately, no specific antiviral medication or treatment is available for enteroviral infection.

ENDEMIC VIRUS

Definition:

Murine typhus [endemic typhus] is a zoonotic disease transmitted by arthropod vector.

Epidemiology:

Urban and suburban areas

Pathophysiology:

The pathogens R.typhi and R.felis are introduced by an arthropod ingesting a blood meal infected with the disease.

Risk factor:

Exposure to arthropod vectors

Symptoms:

Severe headache

Myalgia

Nausea

Vomiting

Diagnosis:

PCR

Treatment:

Antibiotic therapy.

EPILEPSY

Definition:
Epilepsy is a disorder characterized by recurring seizures

Epidemiology:
About 3 million americans have epilepsy

Pathophysiology:
A seizure occurs when too many nerve cells in the brain 'fire' too quickly causing an electrical storm.

Risk factors:
Mental retardation

Cerebral palsy

Stroke

Autism

Symptoms:
Stress

Anxiety

Hormonal changes

Dehydration

Lack of sleep

Extreme fatigue

Photosensitivity

Diagnosis:

Blood tests

EEG

CT

MRI

PET scan

Treatment:

Medication

Surgery

Ketogenic diet

Vagus nerve stimulation.

EPSTEIN – BARR VIRUS INFECTION

Definition:

Infection caused by Epstein-barr virus [EBV]

Epidemiology:

Morethan 95% of worlds population

Pathophysiology:

Infection of the oral epithelial cells cause pharyngitis

Viral replication and cell lysis

Spreads to near structures as salivary glands

Risk factors:

Exposure to virus

Symptoms:

Malaise

Fatigue

Myalgia

Fever

Headache

Sore throat

Nausea

Abdominal pain

Diagnosis:

Heterophilic antibody test

Treatment:

No specific

Acyclovir.

ESOPHAGIAL CANDIADIASIS

Refer candidiasis [disease number 49]

EXTREME COLD [HYPOTHERMIA]

Definition:

Extreme cold conditions

Temperature below 35degree celcius

Epidemiology:

Cool areas

Pathophysiology:

Exposure to cold and cause skin thermoreception and cause shivering, delayed endocrine functions, extrapyramidal stimulation of skeletal muscles

Risk factors:

Radiation

Evaporation

Convection

Conduction

Symptoms:

Vaso constriction

Shivering

Diagnosis:

QT interval prolongation

Sinus bradycardia

Atrial fibrillation

Treatment:

IV fluids should be heated.

Epinephrine, dopamine and other vasoconstrictors should be avoided.

EXTREME HEAT

Definition:

Hyperthermia is a elevated body temperature due to failed thermoregulation.

Epidemiology:

Extreme heat areas

Pathophysiology:

Hyperthermia occurs when the body produces or absorbs more heat that it can dissipate.

Risk factors:

When the elevated body temperature are sufficiently high, heat stroke, environmental exposure to heat.

Symptoms:

Skin may become red

Increased heat dissipation

Tachycardia

Tachypenea

Unconsciousness

Diagnosis:

Physical examination

Body temperature

Treatment:

Anti depressants

Anti cholinergics

Anti histamines

Diuretics

Amphetamines should not be given.

FASCITIS

Definition:

A progressive life threatening sofe tissue infection

Epidemiology:

World wide

Pathophysiology:

Surgery/trauma cause tissue hypoxia and cause dysfunction and necrosis.

Risk factors:

Surgery

Trauma

IM injections

Symptoms:

Purplish skin

Fever

Shock

Diagnosis:

CRP

Leukocytosis

Haemoglobin

Serum sodium

Serum glucose

X ray

MRI

Treatment:

Antibiotics

Surgery

Hyperbaric oxygen therapy [HBO].

FASCIOLA INFECTION

Definition:

Fascioliasis is caused by trematode worms like F.gigantica, F.hepatica.

Epidemiology:

F.gigantica: asia, Africa

F.hepatica: Europe, America, Australia

Pathophysiology:

Free swimming cercariae encyst on water plants, metacercariae on water plant ingested by human, excyst in duodenum and adults in hepatic biliary ducts.

Risk factors:

Farm-level

Symptoms:

Fever

Abdominal pain

GI disturbances

Urticaria

Ascites

Anaemia

Jaundice

Diagnosis:

Fluke eggs in stool

ELISA

Western blot

Treatment:

Triclabendazole

Praziquantel.

FASCIOLOPSIASIS

Refer fasciola infection

FETAL ALCOHOL SPECTRUM DISEASE

Definition:

FASD'S are a group of conditions that occur in a person whose mother drunk alcohol during pregnancy.

Epidemiology:

Mostly US

Pathophysiology:

The effects of alcohol consumption have been shown to cause malformation of vital organs in fetus.

Risk factors:

Pregnant women: consumption of alcohol

Symptoms:

Malformations in fetus vital organs like skeletal, ocular and auditory systems.

Diagnosis:

Examining the fetus

Treatment:

There is no cure and no specific treatment.

FILARIASIS

Definition:

Filariasis is a parasitic disease that is caused by thread-like round worms belonging to filariodea type

Epidemiology:

Worldwide

Pathophysiology:

The pathogenic effect is produced by adult worms of wuchereria, living or dead.

Risk factors:

Those that live in tropical and sub tropical areas

Symptoms:

Edema

Fever

Pruritus

Diagnosis:

Card test

PCR assays

Treatment:

Ivermectin

Albendazole

Diethyl carbamazine.

FLU

Definition:

Flu is a contagious respiratory illness caused by influenza virus,

Epidemiology:

Most commonly encountered deadly disease

Pathophysiology:

When influenza virus is introduced into the respiratory tract by aerosol or by contact with saliva or other respiratory secretions from an infected individual it attaches to and replicates in epithelial cells

Risk factors:

Heart disease

Chronic kidney disease

Diabetes

Obesity

Liver disorders

Anemia

Symptoms:

Sudden onset of high fever

Head ache

Cough

Chills

Sore throat

Nasal congestion

Fatigue

Diagnosis:

Physical examination

Treatment:

Oseltamivir

Zanamivir.

FOLLICULITIS

Definition:

Folliculitis is defined histologically as the presence of inflammatory cells within the wall and ostia of hair follicle, creating a follicular based pustule

Epidemiology:

In the US, superficial folliculitis is quite common

Pathophysiology:

Inflammatory cells within the wall and ostia of the hair follicle, creating a follicular based pustule.

Risk factors:

Trauma

Diabetes mellitus

Immunosuppression

Symptoms:

Redness

Swelling

Pustule formation

Diagnosis:

Physical examination

Treatment:

Weak topical steroids.

FOOD BORNE ILLNESS

Definition:

Illness resulting from consumption of food.

Epidemiology:

Worldwide

Pathophysiology:

Foodborne illness is caused by consuming contaminated foods or beverages.

Risk factors:

Consuming contaminated food

Symptoms:

Vomiting

Diarrhea

Abdominal pain

Fever

Chills

Diagnosis:

Stool examination

Blood cultures

Direct antigen detection tests

Molecular biology techniques

Treatment:

Loperamide

Bismuth subsalicylate.

FRAGILE X SYNDROME

Definition:

Fragile X syndrome that closely associated with gene FMR1 that results in an intellectual disabilities as well as affects physical characteristics of the person.

Epidemiology:

Prevalence estimates for fragile X syndrome vary considerably.

Pathophysiology:

Fragile X syndrome also termed as martin-bell syndrome. It is commonest form of inherited mental retardation.

Risk factors:

Genetics

Symptoms:

Developmental delays

Intellectual and learning disabilities

General or social anxiety

Hyperactivity

Seizures

Depression

Difficulty sleeping

Diagnosis:

DNA blood test

Treatment:

Methylohenidate

Gaunfacine

Clonidine

Selective serotonin reuptake inhibitors.

FRANUCISELLA TULARENSIS INFECTION

Definition:

Tularemia, also known as rabbit fever, is an infectious disease caused by bacterium Francisella tularensis.

Epidemiology:

Tularemia is a zoonotic disease of the northern hemisphere.

Pathophysiology:

Tularemis, is an acute, febrile, granulomatous, infectious zoonosis caused by Francisella tularensis, an aerobic, gram negative, pleomorphic bacillus.

Risk factors:

Frequent contact with animals

Veterinarians

Zookeepers

Parkrangers

Symptoms:

Skin ulcer

Swollen lymph nodes

Severe headaches

Fever

Chills

Fatigue

Diagnosis:

Blood tests

Cultures of infected sites

Treatment:

Streptomycin

Gentamycin

Doxycycline

Ciprofloxacin.

FUNGAL EYE INFECTION

Definition:

Inflammation or infection of the cornea, is known as keratitis and inflammation in the interior of the eye is called endophthalmitis. Many different types of fungi can cause eye infection.

Epidemiology:

The incidence of fungal keratitis has increased over the past 30years

Pathophysiology:

The term fungal keratitis refers to a corneal infection caused by fungi. One type of fungus that can infect the cornea eye is fusarium. When fusarium infects the cornea, the eye disease is referred to as Fusarium keratitis.

Risk factors:

Anyone can get a fungal eye infection.

These infections usually are linked to one of those situaitions: eye surgery or cataract, chronic eye disease involving the surface of the eye.

Symptoms:

Eye pain

Eye redness

Blurred visison

Diagnosis:

Physical examination

Treatment:

Natamycin is a tropical [meaning it is given in the form of eyedrops]

Antifungal medication that works well for fungal infections involving the outer layer of eye particularly those caused by fungi such as aspergillus and fusarium.

FUNGAL MENINGITIS

Definition:

Fungal meningitis is rare and usually caused by fungus spreading through blood to the spinal cord.

Epidemiology:

In the present study, the prevalence of fungal meningitis was noted among 15 [3.1%] of 483AIDS cases. Further, only 2 of 15 cases were females and both acquired HIV infection through blood transfusion.

Pathophysiology:

The most common cause of meningeal inflammation is bacterial or viral infection. Most cases of bacterial meningitis are localized over the dorsum of the brain, however, under certain conditions, meningitis may be concentrated at the base of the brain, as with fungal diseases and tuberculosis.

Risk factors:

Weekened immune system

HIV infection or cancer

Symptoms:

Fever

Headache

Stiff neck

Nausea

Vomiting

Photophobia

Altered mental status

Diagnosis:

If meningitis is suspected, samples of blood or cerebrospinal fluid are collected and sent to a laboratory for testing.

Treatment:

Antifungal medications usually given through an IV in the hospital.

FUNGAL PNEUMONIA

Definition:

Fungal pneumonia is a infection of the lungs by fungi. It can be caused by either endemic or opportunistic fungi or combination of both.

Epidemiology:

Case mortality in fungal pneumonia can be as high as 90% in immunocompromised patients.

Pathophysiology:

Fungi typically enters the lungs with inhalation of their spores, through they can reach the lung through the blood stream if other parts of body are infected also, fungal pneumonia can be caused by reactivation of a latent infection.

Risk factors:

Neutropenic

Symptoms:

Fever

Cough, usually non productive

Pleuritic chestpain

Progressive dyspnea

Airway obstructive symptoms from enlarged mediastinal adenopathy in the endemic mycosis.

Diagnosis:

Chest X ray

[examine lungs]

Treatment:

Administer prophylactic antifungal therapy [i.e treatment with intranasal or IV amphotenem or its other formulations] in patients at high risk for opportunistic fungal infection, including patients with a history of fungal infections.

GAE
[GRANULOMATOUS AMEBIC ENCEPHALITIS]

Definition:

GAE is a central nervous system disease caused by certain species of free living amoeba, especially species of Acanthamoeba and Balamuthia mandrillaris.

Epidemiology:

The disease has a sub acute or chronic onset affecting commonly the immunocompromised population with high mortality rate.

Pathophysiology:

It is rare, usually fatal infection of CNS caused by acanthamoeba species or balamuthia mandrillaris.

Risk factors:

It occurs in people with weekened immune system or generally poor health.

Symptoms:

Confusion

Headache

Seizures

Low grade fever

Blurred vision

Changes in personality

Problem with speaking, coordination and vision.

One side of the body or face may become paralyzed.

Balamuthia mandrillaris may cause skin sores in addition to the symptoms above.

Diagnosis:

CT

MRI

Spinal tap

Treatment:

In one case, cloxacillin, ceftriaxone, amphotericin B were tried. 2 persons were survived after treating successfully with a therapy consisting of flucytosin, pentamidine, fluconazole, sulfadiazine and azithromycin.

GASTROINTESTINAL DISEASES [zoonotic enteric disease]

Definition:

Gastro intestinal infections are viral, bacterial or parasitic infections that cause gastro enteritis.

Epidemiology:

Worldwide

Pathophysiology:

Organ physiology precedes description of organ disease and tightly interwoven into the major sections of disorder and disease in the pathophysiology of their signs, symptoms and laboratory abnormalities.

Risk factors:

Inflammatory bowel disease

Family history

Smoking

NSAID'S

Symptoms:

Acid reflux, heart burn, GERD

Dyspepsia

Nausea

Vomiting

Peptic ulcers disease

Abdominal pain

Belching

Bloating

Flatulence

Biliary tract disorder

Gall bladder disorder

Gall stone pancreatitis

Diagnosis:

Physical condition

Abdominal scan

Treatment:

Antibiotics:

Pencillins

Cephalosporins

Antifolate or sulfa combinations

Nitroimidazole

Penem

Glycopeptide

Monobactum.

GIARDIA INFECTION

Definition:

Giardia infection is an intestinal infection marked by abdominal cramps, bloating, nausea and bouts of watery diarrhea.

Epidemiology:

In the US, it is the most common intestinal parasite disease affecting humans

Pathophysiology:

It is caused by the flagellate protozoan giardia intestinal infection. It is transmitted through ingestion of infectious glamblia cysts. Giardia cysts retain viability in cold water for as long as 2 to 3 months.

Risk factors:

Nail biting

Eating unwashed vegetables raw

Symptoms:

Abdominal pain

Diarrhea

Belching

Bloating

Fat in stool

Indigestion

Nausea

Passing excessive amounts of gas

Fatigue

Loss of appetite

Malaise

Malnutrition

Cramping

Foul smelling stool

Weight loss

Diagnosis:

Stool sample

Treatment:

Metronidazole.

GERMAN MEASELS [RUBELLA VIRUS]

Definition:

It is a contagious viral disease, with symptoms like mild measles. It can cause fetal malformation if caught in early pregnancy.

Epidemiology:

World wide

Pathophysiology:

The usual portal of entry of rubella virus is the respiratory epithelium of the nasopharynx. The virus is transmitted via the aerosol particles from the respiratory tract secretions of infected individuals. The virus attaches and invades the respiratory epithelium.

Risk factors:

Contagious drops of fluid from nose when sneezing and coughing

Symptoms:

Fever

Malaise

Enlarged neck lymphnodes

Eye redness

Red rashes

Runny nose

Diagnosis:

Testing saliva or blood sample

Treatment:

Acetaminophen.

GENITAL WARTS

Definition:

A pointed papilloma typically found on the skin or mucus membranes of the anus and the external genital organs. It is caused by a virus that is transmitted through sexual contact

Epidemiology:

Genital warts are the epidermal manifestations attributed to the epidermotropic human papilloma virus[HPV]

Pathophysiology:

Warts are epidermal manifestations, benign proliferations of the skin and mucosa caused by HPV

Risk factors:

Unprotected sex

Starting sexual relations at young age

Having stress

Sex with many different people

Symptoms:

Painful bumps

Itching

Discharge

Flesh coloured spots

Growths that look like the top of cauliflower.

Diagnosis:

Visual inspection

Treatment:

Cry therapy

Podophyllum

Podofilox cream or gel

Fluorouracil cream

Surgical excision

TCA

Laser therapy

Vitamins and minerals.

GENITAL HERPES

Definition:

Sexually transmitted disease caused by a variety of the herpes simplex virus in which the painful blisters occur in the genital region.

Epidemiology:

Worldwide

Pathophysiology:

HIV-1 infections are spread via respiratory droplets or direct exposure to infected saliva. HIV-2 is usually transmitted via genital contact. The virus travels from the site of infection in the skin or mucosa to sensory dorsal root and remains latent until a recurrent outbreak

Risk factors:

Number of sexual partners in a person's life time

Multiple or frequent changes in a sex partner

Symptoms:

Penis or vaginal pain

Pain during urination

Genital sores

Sensation of pins and needle

Skin rash

Diagnosis:

Viral culture

PCR

Treatment:

Acyclovir

Famiclovir

Valacyclovir.

GENITAL CANDIDIASIS [VULVO VAGINAL CANDIDIASIS]

Definition:

A vaginal yeast infection is a fungal infection that causes irritation, discharge and intense itchness of the vagina and vulva.

Epidemiology:

Millions of the women every year.

Pathophysiology:

Candidiasis is an infection caused by a yeast called candida. Candida normally lives inside the body and on skin without causing any problems.

Risk factors:

Uncontrolled diabetes

Impaired immune system

Corticosteroid therapy

HIV infection

Symptoms:

Pain in the vagina

Pain during sexual intercourse

Vaginal discharge

Vaginal itching

Vaginal inflammation

Vulval inflammation

Redness

Diagnosis:

Gramstain of vaginal discharge]

Treatment:

Intravaginal administration of

Butoconoxole

Clotrimazole

Miconazole

Ticonazole.

GNATHOSTOMA INFECTION

Definition:

Infection caused by gnathostoma [jawed vertebrates]

Epidemiology:

World wide. Most evident in the times of American civil war.

Pathophysiology:

It can hypothesized that the presence of the infectious agents such as dormant mycobacteria

Risk factors:

Low serum albumin concentration

Older age

Obesity

Smoking

Diabetes mellitus

Ischemia

Secondary to vascular disease

Symptoms:

Temperature more than 38 degree Celsius

Skin feels not to touch

Feeling cold or shivering

Aching muscles

Feeling tired

Diarrhea

Headache

Pain when you pass urine

Diagnosis:

Immunological assays

Treatment:

Antibiotics:

Amoxicillin

Ciprofloxacin

Antiviral:

Acyclovir.

GONORRHEA

Definition:

A venereal disease involving inflammatory discharge from the uterus or vagina

Epidemiology:

Gonorrhea is a significant public health problem in the US.

Pathophysiology:

In women, the cervix is the most common site of gonorrhea, resulting in endocervicitis and urethritis, which can be complicated by PID.

In men, gonorrhea causes anterior urithritis

Risk factors:

Sexual activity

Multiple sex partners

Previous history of sexually transmitted disease

Failure to use a condom during sex

Symptoms:

Pain areas: lower abdomen, pelvis, testicle or vagina

Pain circumstances: during intercourse or during urination

Abnormal vaginal discharge

Discharge from penis

Increased vaginal discharge

Irregular menstruation

Diagnosis:

Swabbing the infected site

Treatment:

Antibiotics

Ceftriaxone or cefixime as injection

Azithromycin as tablet.

GOUT

Definition:

A disease in which defective metabolism of uric acid causes arthritis, especially in the smaller bones of the feet, deposition of chalk stones and episodes of acute pain.

Epidemiology:

Most common inflammatory joint disease in men and most common inflammatory arthritis in older women

Pathophysiology:

Gout is caused by monosodium urate monohydrate crystals . pseudogout is caused by calcium pyrophosphate crystals and is more accurately termed calcium pyrophosphate disease.

Risk factors:

Frequent consumptions of food highly in purines including meat, seafood, certain vegetables and beans

Foods containing fructose

Alcohol use

Symptoms:

Pain areas: joints, ankles, foot, knee or toe

Joints: lumps, stiffness, swelling

Physical deformity or redness

Diagnosis:

Use a needle to draw fluid from your affected joint urate crystals may be visible when the fluid is examined under microscope

Treatment:

NSAID'S.

GUILLIAN-BARRE SYNDROME

Definition:

An acute disorder of the peripheral nerves, often preceded by a respiratory infection

Epidemiology:

Worldwide

Pathophysiology:

It is considered to be an auto immune disease triggered by a preceding bacterial or viral infections

Risk factors:

Uncooked food

Poultry

Symptoms:

Pain areas: muscles

Muscle weakness

Fatigue

High blood pressure

Abnormal heart rhythm

Difficulty raising the foot

Difficulty swallowing

Diagnosis:

Lumbar puncture

Treatment:

Plasma exchange

IV immunoglobulin.

GUINEA WORM DISEASE

Definition:

A very long parasitic nematode worm which lives under skin of infected humans and other mammals.

For further information, refer Dracunciliais [disease number 90].

HAB [HARMFUL ALGAL BLOOM ASSOCIATED ILLNESS]

Definition:

HAB composed of phytoplankton known to naturally produce biotoxins. They can occur when certain types of microscopic algae grow quickly in water, forming visible patches that may harm the health of the environment plants or animals.

Epidemiology:

Worldwide

Pathophysiology:

HAB can produce toxins that have caused a variety of illness in people and animals

Risk factors:

Contaminated drinking water

Symptoms:

Rash

Blisters

Cough

Wheezing

Congestion

Sore throat

Ear ache

Eye irritation

Diagnosis:

Microscopic images

Molecular biology techniques

Treatment:

Cost effective.

HANSEN'S DISEASE

Definition:

Also known as Leprosy

A chronic, curable infectious disease mainly causing skin lesions and nerve damage

Epidemiology:

Worldwide

Pathophysiology:

Leprosy is a chronic infection caused by the acid fast, rod shaped bacillus Mycobacterium leprae. Leprosy can be considered to be 2 connected diseases that primarily affect superficial tissues, especially the skin and the peripheral nerves. Initially a mycobacterial infection causes a wide array of cellular immune responses.

Risk factors:

Weekened immune systems

Diabetes

HIV

AIDS

Heart diseases

Symptoms:

Pain: joints

Skin: blister, loss of colour, rashes, ulcers, redness

Reduced sensation of touch

Nerve injury

Weight loss

Diagnosis:

Skin or nerve biopsy
Acid fast staining

Treatment:

Combination of antibiotics

Dapsone with rifampicin

Clofaximine is added for some types of the disease.
This is called multidrug therapy.

HANTAVIRUS PULMONARY SYNDROME [HPS]

Definition:

It is a febrile illness characterized by bilateral interstitial pulmonary infiltrates and respiratory compromise usually requiring supplemental oxygen and clinically resembling acute respiratory disease syndrome [ARDS]

Epidemiology:

First discovered in north America

Pathophysiology:

The pathophysiology of pulmonary findings is that of pulmonary capillary leak syndrome. Hantavirus particles are found within the renal tubular cells of patients with HPS.

Risk factors:

Inhaling infected rodent urine

Dropping or saliva

Presence of infected rodents in and around the home environment

Symptoms:

Pain areas: abdomen, chest, muscles

Fever

Chills

Fatigue

Malaise

Low BP

Diarrhea

Nausea

Vomiting

Shortness of breath

Fluid in the lungs

Headache

Cough

Diagnosis:

Physical examination

Treatment:

The nucleoside analogue ribavirin has been shown to be effective in hemorrhage fever with renal failure syndrome caused by hantavirus.

HEARING IMPAIRMENT

Definition:

Hearing loss, also known as hearing impairment, is a partial or total inability to hear

Epidemiology:

The prevalence of mild hearing impairment are worse [less than 20 db] is 3.1% based on the average audiometric screening studies

Pathophysiology:

Results from anything that decreases the transmission of sound from the outside world to cochlea. Sounds perceived by the brain and diminished but are generally not distorted. Sensorineural hearing loss may result from disruptions in transmission after the cochlea

Risk factors:

Exposed to loud noise

Symptoms:

Hearing problems

Ringing in the ears

Sensitivity to sound

Social isolation

Speech delay in a child

Diagnosis:

Self diagnosable

Treatment:

Treatment can help, but this condition can't be cured.

HEARTLAND VIRUS INFECTION

Definition:

Infection caused by heartland virus, a tick borne phlebovirus.

Epidemiology:

More in US.

Pathophysiology:

Infection

Risk factors:

Exposure to virus

Symptoms:

Fever

Headache

Muscle pain

Loss of appetite

Nausea

Diarrhea

Weight loss

Jointpain

Leucopenia

Thrombocytopenia

Diagnosis:

RT-PCR

Treatment:

IV Fluids.

HEAT STRESS

Refer hypothermia [disease number 104]

HEMOPHILIA AND BLOOD RELATED DISORDERS

Definition:

Hemophilia is a most inherited genetic disorder that impairs the body's ability to make blood clots

Epidemiology:

Worldwide

Pathophysiology:

Hemophilia A is caused by mutation in the gene for factor 8, so there is deficiency of this clotting factor.

Hemophilia B results from a deficiency of factor 9 due to mutation in the corresponding gene

Risk factors:

Congenital

Symptoms:

Hematuria

Nausea

Vomiting

Lethargy

Diagnosis:

Clotting time

Treatment:

Use of factor replacement products and other medications including pain medications is typically required.

HENDRA VIRUS DISEASE

Definition:

Hendra virus: a virus carried by bats which is potentially fatal to animals and humans.

Epidemiology:

World wide

Pathophysiology:

Hendravirus and niphavirus are emerging zoonotic viruses that cause severe and often lethal respiratory illness and encephalitis in humans

Risk factors:

Contact with live pig

Symptoms:

Fever

Cough

Sore throat

Headache

Tiredness

Diagnosis:

ELISA

RT-PCR

Treatment:

There is no cure, specific treatment or human vaccine for Hendra virus.

HEPATITIS A AND B

HEPATITIS A

Definition:

A form of viral hepatitis transmitted in food, causing fever and jaundice

Epidemiology:

Worldwide

Pathophysiology:

Hepatitis virus [HAV] is a single stranded, positive sense, linear RNA enterovirus of picornaviridae family. In humans, viral replication depends on hepatocyte uptake and synthesis, assembly occurs exclusively in liver cells. No antibody cross reactivity has been identified with other virus causing acute hepatitis.

Risk factors:

WHO has not been vaccinated

Previously infected

Symptoms:

Fatigue

Nausea

Abdominal pain

Loss of appetite

Low grade fever

Dark urine

Weight loss

Diagnosis:

Blood test

Treatment:

Agents used include:

Analgesics

Anti emetics

Vaccines

Immunoglobulins

Acetaminophen dose should not be more than 4gram per day.

HEPATITIS B

Definition:

It is a serious disease caused by a virus that infects the liver

Epidemiology:

1/3rd of worlds population has been infected

Pathophysiology:

HBV via cell mediated immune response cause mild symptoms and may result in chronic disease.

Risk factors:

Injection drug users

Sex partners of those hepB

Sex with morethan one partner

Transfusions

Travel

Dialysis

Symptoms:

Nausea

Loss of appetite

Vomiting

Fatigue

Fever

Dark urine

Pale stools

Jaundice

Stomach pain

Side pain

Diagnosis:

HBS-ag

HBV – DNA

Treatment:

Interferon alpha

Lamivudine

Adefovir

Tenofovir

Entecavir.

HISTOPLASMOSIS

Definition:

Infection by a fungus found in the droppings of birds and bats in humid areas

Epidemiology:

Worldwide

Pathophysiology:

Inhale spores affects the lymph nodes, liver, spleen, adrenal glands, intestine, bone marrow.

Risk factors:

Farmers

Pest control workers

Poultry keepers

Cave explorers

Symptoms:

Fever

Chills

Headache

Muscle aches

Dry cough

Chest discomfort

Diagnosis:

Sputum test

Blood test

Urine test

Treatment:

Antifungal

NSAID'S.

HIV

Refer AIDS

Disease number 4

HYPERTENSION

Definition:

Condition in which the flow of blood against the artery wall is too high

Epidemiology:

Between 10 and 25% of population are expected to benefit from drug treatment of hypertension

Pathophysiology:

Arterial pressure causes changes in cardiac output and heartrate and finally leads to changes in the size of vascular component and myocardial contractility, changes in vascular structure and functioning.

Risk factors:

Lack of physical activities

Being obese

Unhealthy diet

Drinking too much of alcohol

Sleep apnea

High cholesterol diet

Diabetes

Smoking

Family history

Symptoms:

Asymptomatic

Diagnosis:

Via sphygmomanometer

Treatment:

Angiotension convertase inhibitors

Angiotension receptor blockers

Diuretics

Calcium channel blockers

Beta adrenoceptor antagonists

Alpha adrenoceptor blockers

Centrally acting agents

Directly acting vasodilators.

HYPOTENSION

Definition:

Any blood pressure that is below the normal expected for an individual in given environment.

Epidemiology:

Worldwide

Pathophysiology:

Changes in cardiac output [lower] leads to arrhythmia, hypovolemia, systemic vasodilation and finally hypotension.

Risk factors:

Reduced cardiac output

Hypovolemia

Vascular obstruction

Symptoms:

Feeling lightheadedness

Blurry vision

Weakness

Fainting

Confusion

Nausea

Diagnosis:

Sphygmomanometer

Treatment:

Fluorocortisone

Midrodrine.

HPIV [HUMAN PARA INFLUENZA VIRUS]

Definition:

They are the second most common cause of lower respiratory tract infection, especially in younger children.

Epidemiology:

These are common community acquired respiratory pathogens

Pathophysiology:

HPIV infection in the respiratory tract leads to secretion of high levels of inflammatory cytokines.

Risk factors:

Bronchitis

Bronchiolitis

Pneumonia

Symptoms:

Nasal congestion

Runny nose

Sore throat

Cough

Inflammation of nasal cavity

Diagnosis:

Pulse oximetry

Laryngoscopy

Radiography

Treatment:

Analgesics

Ribavirin

Corticosteroids

Nebulized epinephrine.

HANTAVIRUS PULMONARY SYNDROME [HPS]

Refer disease 133

HUMAN PAPILLOMAVIRUS INFECTION [HPV]

Definition:

Anogenital disease

Cervical / vaginal / vulvar / anal / penile

Epidemiology:

Worldwide

Pathophysiology:

Invasion of the virus into anogenital areas

Risk factors:

Genital contact

Smoking

Alcohol consumption

Number of sexual partners

Symptoms:

Head or neck disease

Cancer

Diagnosis:

HPV test

Treatment:

Antibody titers.

IMPETIGO

Definition:

Impetigo is a superficial skin infection that is seen most commonly in children and is transmitted easily from person to person.

Epidemiology:

Low-middle income countries

Pathophysiology:

On exposed skin, superficial erosion and a yellow crust

Risk factors:

Transmitted through:

Towels

Toys

Clothing

Symptoms:

Severe itching

Weakness

Fever

Diarrhea

Regional lymph nodes may be enlarged

Diagnosis:

Physical examination

Complete blood count

Culture test

Treatment:

Ointment mupirocin

Anti microbial treatment

Pencillin

Cefadroxil

Clindamycin.

INFECTIOUS MONONUCLEOSIS

Refer Epstein-barr virus [disease number 102]

INFERTILITY

Definition:

Inability to conceive after 12 months of having sexual intercourse with average frequency [2 to 3 times per week] without the use of any form of birth control.

Epidemiology:

Average incidence of infertility is about 15% globally.

Pathophysiology:

1 time per week : 17% probability of conception

3 times per week : 50% probability of conception

Risk factors:

Leprosy

Gonorrhea

Chlamydia

Tuberculosis

Mumps

Age more than 40 years

Smoking

Alcohol

Symptoms:

Women:

Endocrinopathy

Congenital anomalies

Uterine hypoplasia

Cervical lesions

Men:

Hypogonadism

Tumors

Epididymal cysts

Diagnosis:

Female:

Urine test

Basal body temperature

Hysteroscopy

Endometrial biopsy

Male:

Semen count

Urine analysis

Endocrine test

Treatment:

Ovulation inducing drugs

Surgical procedures

IU insemination.

INFLAMMATORY BOWEL DISEASE

Definition:

Ongoing inflammation of all or part of the digestive tract

Types:

Ulcerative colitis:

Chronic inflammatory bowel disease that causes inflammation in the digestive tract.

Crohn's disease

Refer disease number 77.

INFLUENZA

Refer disease number 111 [flu]

INTESTINAL AMEBIC INFECTION

Refer amoebiasis [disease number 11]

JAPANESE ENCEPHALITIS

Definition:

A mosquito borne flavor virus infection that is leading cause of viral encephalitis in asia. Japanese encephalitis virus cannot be transmitted from person to person

Epidemiology:

Tropical regions of asia

Japan

Pathophysiology:

Virus inters into body through bite of insect vector

Virus is transported to target organ via blood

Virus proliferate and damage the neuronal tissue, thereby elicits nervous manifestations.

Risk factors:

Summer season

Outdoor recreational activities

Contact with mosquitoes, birds, pigs

Symptoms:

Fever

Head ache

Vomiting

Mental status changes

Diagnosis:

CSF

Treatment:

Anti pyretics

Anti convulsants

Treatment of secondary bacterial infection

Maintenance of nutrition.

JAUNDICE

Definition:

It is the yellowish discolouration of the tissues due to deposition of bilirubin which occurs in presence of hyperbilirubinemia.

Epidemiology:

10% of population experience this at anytime of their life

Pathophysiology:

Increased bilirubin load secondary to increased RBC volume, decreased RBC life span, or increased enterohepatic circulation.

Risk factors:

Malaria

Sickle cell disease

Thalassemia

Drugs or other toxins

Symptoms:

Pale coloured stools

Dark coloured urine

Skin itching

Nausea and vomiting

Rectal bleeding

Diarrhea

Head ache

Diagnosis:

Physical examination

Blood test

Urine test

Treatment:

Light therapy

IV immunoglobulin

Exchange transfusion.

KAWASAKI DISEASE

Definition:

Also known as Kawasaki syndrome

Mucocutaneous lymphnode syndrome

Epidemiology:

Worldwide

Pathophysiology:

Involves the skin, mouth and lymph nodes

Inflammation of blood vessels

Risk factors:

80% of children under the age of 5

Symptoms:

High fever

Red eyes

Sore throat

Swollen lymphnodes

Swollen painful joints

Vomiting

Diarrhea

Abdominal pain

Diagnosis:

There is no specific test

Treatment:

Aspirin therapy

Gamma globulin IV.

KERATITIS

Definition:

Inflammation of the cornea of the eye

Epidemiology:

2 to 11 per 1,00,000 per year

Pathophysiology:

Inflammation of the cornea, the transparent dome-like portion of eyeball in front of iris and pupil due to microorganisms

Risk factors:

Trauma

Contact lens use

Pre existing ocular disease

Exposure to pathogens

Symptoms:

Eyepain

Blurred vision

Photophobia

Tearing

Eye redness

Diagnosis:

By use of slit lamp

Treatment:

Bacterial keratitis : anti bacterial eyedrops

Fungal keratitis : anti fungal eyedrops

Viral keratitis : anti viral eyedrops

Acanthamoeba keratitis: antibiotic eyedrops.

KYASANUR FOREST DISEASE [KFD]

Definition:

KFD is a tick-borne viral hemorrhagic fever

Epidemiology:

Endemic to south asia

Pathophysiology:

Kyasanur forest disease virus and alkhurma hemorrhage fever virus are genetically closely related

Risk factors:

Exposure

Symptoms:

Abnormal low blood pressure

Low platelet, RBC, WBC count

Fever

Severe headache

Mental disturbances

Tremors

Vision deficits

Diagnosis:

PCR

ELISA

Treatment:

No specific treatment

Supportive therapy must be given.

KIDNEY DISEASE

Definition:

Slowing the progression of kidney

Epidemiology:

Causes morethan 95,000 deaths a year

Pathophysiology:

Inherited kidney disorders

Congenital kidney diseases

Acquired kidney diseases

Risk factors:

High blood pressure

Diabetes

Smoking

Obesity

Family history

Symptoms:

Nausea

Vomiting

Loss of appetite

Fatigue

Sleep problems

Muscle cramps

Chest pain

Shortness of breath

High bloodpressure

Diagnosis:

Blood tests

Urine tests

Imaging tests

Removing a sample of kidney tissue for testing

Treatment:

Treat symptoms

Dialysis

Kidney transplant.

LA CROSSE ENCEPHALITIS

Definition:

LACV is one of the group of mosquito transmitted viruses that can cause encephalitis or inflammation of the brain

Epidemiology:

80 to 100 cases each year in US

Pathophysiology:

Caused by arbovirus

Risk factors:

Exposure

Symptoms:

Fever

Headache

Nausea

Vomiting

Tiredness

Diagnosis:

Blood test

Spinal fluid test

Treatment:

Hospitalization

Respiratory support

IV fluids.

LASSA FEVER

Definition:

Viral hemorrhagic fever caused by Arenavirus lassa

Epidemiology:

Endemic in portions of west asia

Pathophysiology:

Rodent to human

Human to human

Endothelial cell damage

Platelet dysfunction

Suppressed cardiac function

Risk factors:

Exposure to virus

Symptoms:

Hemorrhaging : gums, nose, eyes

Breathing

Cough

Swollen airways

Diarrhea

Tremors

Diagnosis:

ELISA

RT-PCR

Virus isolation

Treatment:

Ribavirin.

LATEX ALLERGIES

Definition:

Allergic reactions to latex may be serious and can very rarely be fatal.

Epidemiology:

Worldwide

Pathophysiology:

Allergic reactions to products made with latex develop in persons who become allergic to proteins contained in natural rubber latex

Risk factors:

Exposure to latex products

Symptoms:

Itching

Stuffy nose

Asthma symptoms

Anaphylaxis

Shock

Diagnosis:

Physical examination

Blood tests

Treatment:

No specific treatment

Treat symptoms

Avoid latex products.

LYMPHOCYTIC CHORIOMENINGITIS

Definition:

LCM is a rodent borne viral disease.

Epidemiology:

5% of population

Pathophysiology:

LCMV infections can occur after exposure to fresh urine, droppings, saliva or nesting materials from infected rodents.

Risk factors:

Individuals of all ages who come into contact with urine, feces, saliva or blood of wild mice

Laboratory workers

Symptoms:

Fever

Malaise

Loss of appetite

Muscle aches

Headache

Nausea

Vomiting

Joint pain

Diagnosis:

IgM and IgG antibodies in CSF and serum

PCR

Virus isolation

Treatment:

Anti inflammatory drugs

Corticosteroids

Ribavirin.

LEGIONELLOSIS:

Definition:

A series and sometimes fatal form of pneumonia, caused by Legionella pneumophilia.

Epidemiology:

Among the 182 infected patients, 147 were hospitalized and 29 died.

Pathophysiology:

Inhalation of contaminated water sources

Association with travel

Risk factors:

Smokers

Immune deficient people

Patients on immune suppression drugs

Symptoms:

Feeling tired

High fever

Cough

GI symptoms

Head ache

Muscle ache

Diagnosis:

Urinary antigen test

Chest X ray

Treatment:

Macrolides:

Azithromycin

Fluoroquinolones:

Moxifloxacin.

LEISHMANIA INFECTION

Definition:

Leishmaniasis is a globally important but neglected disease

Epidemiology:

2 million people every year

Pathophysiology:

Fly bites human

Risk factors:

Pet owners

Symptoms:

Symptoms depend on the form of disese

Cutaneous

Muco cutaneous

Visceral

Diagnosis:

Smear

Biopsy

Treatment:

Antiparasitic drugs such as amphotericin B.

LEPROSY

Refer Hansen's disease [disease number 132]

LOA-LOA INFECTION

Definition:

Loa loa is a blood dwelling nematode that is parasitic to human beings

Epidemiology:

Topical, central and west Africa

Pathophysiology:

Transmitted by bite of an infected deerfly

Risk factors:

Who lives in west and central Africa

Symptoms:

Swelling near joints

Worms crawling across the eyes

Muscle and joint pain

Tiredness and fatigue

Diagnosis:

Examining sample of blood under microscope

Treatment:

Chemotherapy

Surgical removal of adult worms.

LOUSE BORNE RELAPSING FEVER

Definition:

LBRF is a vector borne disease

Epidemiology:

10 to 40 percent death

2 to 5 percent treated patients

Pathophysiology:

Caused by spirochaete borellia recurrentis

Risk factors:

Exposure

Symptoms:

High fever

Malaise

Chills

Sweats

Headache

Myalgia

GI symptom

Hepatomegaly

Splenomegaly

Diagnosis:

Identification of spirochaetes in blood

Treatment:

Antibiotics:

Tetracycline

Pencillin G

Erythromycin

Chloramphenicol.

LUNG CANCER

Definition:

Lung carcinoma, is a malignant lung tumor characterized by controlled cell growth in tissues of lung.

Epidemiology:

About 14% of all new cancers are lung cancers

Pathophysiology:

Uncontrolled cell growth in tissues of the lungs

Risk factors:

Tobacco smoke

Exposure to asbestos

Talc and talcum powder

Symptoms:

Cough with sputum

Chest pain

Hemoptysis

Hoarseness

Weight loss

Loss of appetite

Shortness of breath

Diagnosis:

Complete blood count

Chest X ray

CT

PET scan

Bronchoscopy

Treatment:

Laser therapy

Chemotherapy

Cisplatin

Carboplatin

Taxol

Docetaxel

Vinblastine.

LYME DISEASE

Definition:

It is also known as Lyme borreliosis, is an infectious disease caused by bacteria of borellia type which spread of ticks

Epidemiology:

Mostly in US

Pathophysiology:

Infectious disease

Spread by ticks

Risk factors:

Exposure to ticks

Field workers

Symptoms:

Expanding areas of redness at the site of tick bite

Fever

Headache

Feeling tired

Diagnosis:

Based on symptoms

Blood test

Treatment:

Doxycycline

Amoxicillin

Cefuroxime.

LYMPHEDEMA

Definition:

Lymphedema is swelling in one or more extremities that results from impaired flow of lymphatic system

Epidemiology:

Worldwide

Pathophysiology:

Swelling of one or more extremities that results from impaired flow of lymphatic system

Risk factors:

Abnormalities of lymph vessels

Symptoms:

Decreased ability to see or feel the veins or tendons in the extremities

Redness of the skin

Slight puffiness of the skin

Fever

Chills

Diagnosis:

CT

MRI

Ultrasound scan

Treatment:

Treat the symptoms.

MAD COW DISEASE

Refer bovine spongiform encephalopathy [disease
number 39]

MALARIA

Definition:

Malaria is a mosquito borne infectious disease affecting humans and other animals caused by parasitic protozoans.

Epidemiology:

Worldwide

Pathophysiology:

Plasmodium spread by mosquitoes

Risk factors:

Exposure to mosquitoes

Symptoms:

Fever

Tiredness

Vomiting

Headaches

Yellow skin

Seizures

Coma

Death

Diagnosis:

Examination of the blood

Antigen detection tests

Treatment:

Pyremethamine

Artemesin

Mefloquine

Quinine + doxycycline.

MARBURG HEMORRHAGIC FEVER

Definition:

Marburg hemorrhagic fever is a rare, severe type of hemorrhagic fever which affects both humans and non-human primates

Epidemiology:

It is indigenous to Africa

Pathophysiology:

Just how the animal host first transmits Marburg virus to humans is unknown

Risk factors:

Droplets to bodyfluids

Direct contact with person

Symptoms:

Fever

Chills

Head ache

Myalgia

Rash

Sore throat

Pancreatitis

Liver failure

Diagnosis:

PCR

ELISA

Virus isolation

Treatment:

No specific treatment

Fluids

Electrolytes.

MUSCULAR DYSTROPHY

Definition:

Muscular dystrophy refers to a group of disorders that involve a progressive loss of muscle mass and consequent loss of strength.

Epidemiology:

1 in every 5000 males

Pathophysiology:

Caused by genetic mutations

Risk factors:

Increased age

Sex : male

Family history

Symptoms:

Pain and stiffness in the muscles

Difficulty with running and jumping

Learning disabilities

Frequent falls

Inability to walk

Symptoms:

Based on symptoms

Treatment:

Corticosteroids

Beta blockers

Angiotension convertase inhibitors.

MEASLES

Definition:

Measles is a highly contagious infectious disease caused by measles virus

Epidemiology:

Approximately 73,400 deaths every year

Pathophysiology:

Infection caused by virus

Risk factors:

Exposure to virus

Symptoms:

Fever

Cough

Runny nose

Inflamed eyes

Rash

Diagnosis:

Based on symptoms

Treatment:

Acetaminophen

Rest

Plenty of fluids

Humidifier

Vitamin A supplements.

MENINGITIS

Definition:

Meningitis is an acute inflammation of the protective membranes covering the brain and spinal cord, known collectively as the meninges.

Epidemiology:

Approximately 3,79,000 every year worldwide

Pathophysiology:

Viral

Bacteria

Other

Risk factors:

Exposure to virus, bacteria

Symptoms:

Fever

Headache

Neck stiffness

Diagnosis:

Blood cultures

CT

MRI

X rays

Spinal tap

Treatment:

Bacterial : IV antibiotics

        Corticosteroids

Viral : antiviral

        Corticosteroids.

MENTAL RETARDATION

Definition:

It is a generalizes neuro development disorder characterized by significantly impaired intellectual and adaptive functioning.

Epidemiology:

Affects 2 to 3 % of general population

Pathophysiology:

Overall intelligent quotient lower than 70

Risk factors:

IQ levels

Genetic

Symptoms:

Delays in oral language development

Deficits in memory skills

Difficulty learning

Decreased learning ability

Lack of social inhibition

IQ lower than 70

Diagnosis:

Based on symptoms

IQ levels

Treatment:

No cure

Appropriate guidance.

MICROCEPHALY

Definition:

It is a rare neurological condition in which an infant's head is significantly smaller.

Epidemiology:

Worldwide

Pathophysiology:

Developmental issues

Risk factors:

Genetics

Malnutrition

Environmental factors

Chromosomal abnormalities

Symptoms:

A head size significantly smaller than that of other children of same age and sex.

Diagnosis:

Head size is measured

Treatment:

No treatment

Supportive therapies:

Speech and occupational therapies.

MICRONUTRIENT MALNUTRITION

Definition:

Defined as lack of essential vitamins and minerals required in small amounts by the body for proper growth and development.

Epidemiology:

Worldwide

Pathophysiology:

Lack of essential vitamins and minerals

Risk factors:

Pregnant women

Children

Symptoms:

Vitamin deficiencies

Anaemia

Scurvy

Diagnosis:

Based on physical examination

Treatment:

Supplementation of vitamins and minerals
Food fortification
Biofortification.

MICROSPORODIA INFECTION

Definition:

Infection caused by microsporidia

Intestinal infection

Epidemiology:

Worldwide

Pathophysiology:

Infection caused by microsporidia, which are spore forming parasites

Risk factors:

Ingestion or inhalation of microsporidia spores

Symptoms:

Diarrhea

Malabsorption

Gallbladder disease

Eye infections

UTI

Diagnosis:

Microscopic examination of stained samples

PCR

Treatment:

Albendazole

IV Fluid.

MIDDLE EAST RESPIRATORY SYNDROME CORONAVIRUS

Refer covid-19

MONKEY POX

Definition:

Monkey pox is an infectious disease caused by monkey pox virus.

Epidemiology:

The disease mostly occurs in central and west Africa.

Pathophysiology:

Virus entry

Risk factors:

Exposure to virus

Symptoms:

Head ache

Muscle pains

Blistering rash

Swollen lymph nodes

Diagnosis:

Testing for viral DNA

Treatment:

Currently, there is no proven, safe treatment for monkey pox. The people who have been infected can be vaccinated upto 14 days after exposure.

MULTIPLE ORGAN DYSFUNCTION SYNDROME

Definition:

MODS is altered o.rgan function is an acutely illpatient requiring medical intervention to achieve homeostasis.

Epidemiology:

Worldwide

Pathophysiology:

Local and systemic responses are initiated by tissue damage.

Risk factors:

Stroke patients

Hypertension patients

Symptoms:

Multiple organ dysfunction

Diagnosis:

Sepsis-related organ failure assessment [SOFA] score to describe and quantitate the degree of organ dysfunction in 6 organ systems.

Treatment:

Antimicrobial therapy

Vasopressor therapy

Norepinephrine

Epinephrine

Dopamine

Corticosteroidal therapy.

MUMPS

Definition:

Mumps is a viraldisease caused by mumps virus

Epidemiology:

Worldwide

Pathophysiology:

Contagious disease

Condition primarily affects the salivary glands

Risk factors:

Exposure to virus

Contact with the person having mumps

Symptoms:

Fatigue

Body aches

Head ache

Loss of appetite

Low grade fever

Diagnosis:

Virus culture

Blood test

Treatment:

Rest in bed

Isolate yourself

Acetaminophen

NSAID'S

Drink plenty of fluid.

MURINE TYPHUS

Refer endemic typhus [disease number 100]

MYCOBACTERIUM AVIUM COMPLEX [MAC]

Definition:

MAC, is a type of bacterial infection that can cause life threatening symptoms in people who have compromised immune systems.

Epidemiology:

MAC organisms can be found virtually anywhere in the environment.

Pathophysiology:

Infection caused by bacteria

Risk factors:

Exposure to bacteria

AIDS

Diarrhea

Malabsorption

Symptoms:

Fever – main symptom

Night sweats

Chills

Weight loss

Muscle wasting

Abdominal pain

Fatigue

Diagnosis:

Blood or bone marrow samples are collected and sent to a lab for testing

Treatment:

Clarithromycin

Ethambutol

Rifabutin

Amikacin

Streptomycin.

MYIASIS

Definition:

Myiasis is the parasitic infestation of the body of a live mammal by fly larvae [maggots] that grow inside the host while feeding on it's tissue.

Epidemiology:

Worldwide

Pathophysiology:

Parasitic infestion of body of live mammal by maggots that grow inside the host while feeding on it's tissue.

Risk factors:

Poor hygiene

Poor sanitary conditions

Advanced age

Psychiatric illness

Alcoholism

Diabetes

Vascular disease

Symptoms:

Cutaneous myiasis

Nasal myiasis

Opthalmomyiasis

Boils

Vision abnormalities

Diarrhea

Vomiting

Diagnosis:

Blood test

MRI

Ultrasound

Biopsy

Treatment:

Anthelminthics.

MYDRIASIS

Definition:

Dilation of the pupil of the eye

Epidemiology:

Worldwide

Pathophysiology:

Sympathetic stimulation of the adrenergic receptors cause the contraction of the radial muscle and subsequent dilation of pupil.

Risk factors:

Diabetes mellitus

Eye trauma

Symptoms:

Dilation of pupil

Sensitivity to light

Diagnosis:

Physical examination

Treatment:

Light sensitive sunglasses

Opaque contact lenses

Surgery.

NAEGLERIA INFECTION

Definition:

It is the infection caused by Naegleria floweris known as 'brain-eating amoeba'

Epidemiology:

Rare

Pathophysiology:

Invasion of the blood stream

Retrograde neuronal pathway

Direct contagious speed

Risk factors:

Exposure occurs during swimming or other water spots

Symptoms:

A change in the sense of smell and taste

Fever

Sudden, severe headache

Stiffness

Sensitivity to light

Nausea

Sleepiness

Seizures

Diagnosis:

Physical examination

CSF analysis

Treatment:

Amphotericin B

Adjunctive therapy:

Fluconazole

Azithromycin

Rifampin.

NACROVIRUS INFECTION

Refer CCHF

NEUROCYSTICERCOSIS

Definition:

It is a specific form of infectious parasitic disease cysticercosis.

Epidemiology:

50 to 100 million people infected worldwide

Pathophysiology:

The cestode Taenia solium is the main cause of main cause of human cysticercosis.

Risk factors:

Exposure to Taenia solium

Symptoms:

Seizures

Headache

Nausea

Abdominal cramps

Diagnosis:

Physical examination

Serology

Brain imaging

Treatment:

Anti epileptic drugs

Corticosteroids

Anthelminthic drugs.

NOCARDIOSIS

Definition:

Nocardiosis is a disease caused by bacteria found in soil and water. It can affect the lungs, brain, and skin

Epidemiology:

All age groups

Worldwide

Pathophysiology:

Infection via inhalation or by direct inoculation of the skin'

Risk factors:

Organ transplantation

High dose corticosteroid

Underlying pulmonary disease

Symptoms:

Cough

Fever

Chills

Chestpain

Weakness

Anorexia

Weight loss

Diagnosis:

Cultures of sample

X ray

Imaging

Treatment:

Trimethoprim/sulfamethoxazole

NOROVIRUS INFECTION

Definition:

Norovirus is a very contagious virus that can infect anyone

Epidemiology:

Worldwide

Pathophysiology:

Infection caused by virus

Risk factors:

Exposure to virus

Symptoms:

Vomiting

Watery diarrhea

Stomach pain

Diagnosis:

Stool sample

Treatment:

No specific treatment

Give vitamins and supplements.

OSTEOARTHRITIS

Definition:

It is a joint disease caused by cartilage loss in a joint.

Epidemiology:

Worldwide

Pathophysiology:

Cartilage loss

Risk factors:

Previous joint injury

Abnormal joint

Inherited factors

Symptoms:

Joint pain

Stiffness

Joint swelling

Decreased range of motion

Diagnosis:

X-ray

MRI

Blood tests

Joint fluid analysis

Treatment:

Acetaminophen

NSAID'S

Cortisone injections

Lubrication injections

Joint replacement

Life style modifications.

OBESITY

Definition:

Obesity is a medical condition in which excess body fat has accumulated to the extent that it may have a negative effect on health.

Epidemiology:

Worldwide

Pathophysiology:

Excess body fat accumulation

Risk factors:

Excessive food

Lack of exercise

Genetics

Symptoms:

Increased fat

Inability to walk for sometime

Diagnosis:

BMI more than 30kg/m square

Treatment:

Diet

Exercise

Medication

Surgery.

OCCUPATIONAL CANCER

Refer cancer

OHF [OMSK HEMORRHAGIC FEVER]

Definition:

OHF is a viral hemorrhagic fever caused by flavivirus

Epidemiology:

Found in Siberia

Pathophysiology:

Fever caused by flavivirus originates in ticks, who then transmit it to rodents by biting them. Human become infected through tick bites

Risk factors:

Tick bites

Contact with infected blood, feces, urine of dead or sick musk rat

Symptoms:

Chills

Headache

Pain in the lower and upper extremitis

A rash on the soft palate

Swollen glands in the neck

GI symptoms

CNS symptoms

Diagnosis:

Serological testing using immunosorbent serological assay

Treatment:

No specific treatment

Supportive therapy.

ORAL CANCER

Definition:

Oral cancer, also known as mouth cancer, is a type of head and neck cancer and is any cancerous tissue growth located in the oral cavity

Epidemiology:

Oral cancer occurs more often in people from the lower end of the socioeconomic scale.

Pathophysiology:

Abnormal growth of cells

Cancerous tissue growth

Mutation of DNA

Risk factors:

Tobacco use

Alcohol consumption

Poor oral hygiene

Bacterial or viral infections

Symptoms:

Persistent red or white patches

Non healing ulcer

Unusual surface changes

Unusual oral bleeding

Paresthesia

Otalgia

Diagnosis:

X ray

CT

MRI

Tissue biopsy

Treatment:

Surgery

Radiation

Chemotherapy

Targeted drug therapy.

ORF VIRUS INFECTION

Definition:

Orf is a viral skin disease that can be spread to humans by handling infected sheep and goats

Epidemiology:

Morbidity may reach 100% and fatality rate 5% to 15%

Pathophysiology:

Disease caused by parapoxvirus

Risk factors:

Farmers

Butches

People with weekend immune system

Symptoms:

Small, red, itchy, painful lump

Mild fever

General tiredness

Enlarged lymph glands

Diagnosis:

Diagnosis is based on characteristic lesions.

Treatment:

No specific treatment

Imiquimod cream.

OROYA FEVER

Refer Bartonella bacillifornis infection which is also called carrion's disease

OTITIS

Definition:

Otitis media is a group of inflammatory disease of the middle ear

Epidemiology:

Worldwide

Pathophysiology:

The cause is related to childhood anatomy and immune function. Inflammation occurs in the ear.

Risk factors:

Exposure to smoke

Attending day care

Viral

Bacterial

Symptoms:

Earpain

Fever

Hearing loss

Diagnosis:

Looking at the eardrum

Treatment:

Paracetamol

Ibuprofen

Benzocaine

Amoxicillin.

OVARIAN CANCER

Definition:

Ovarian cancer is a type of cancer that begins in the ovaries

Epidemiology:

14,000 deaths from the condition each year

Pathophysiology:

Abnormal growth of cells leads to cancer

Risk factors:

Menstrual cycles

Family history

Women

IVF

Symptoms:

Fatigue

Abdominal swelling

Clothes suddenly not fitting

Abdominal pain

Shortness of breath

Diagnosis:

Screening tests

Pelvic or abdominal ultrasound

X ray

CT scans

Biopsy

Treatment:

Surgical treatment

Chemotherapy

Targeted therapy: avastin.

PERIPHERAL ARTERIAL DISEASE

Definition:

PAD is a common condition, in which a build-up of fatty deposits in the arteries restricts blood supply to leg muscles. It is known as peripheral vascular disease

Epidemiology:

Worldwide

Pathophysiology:

Build-up of fatty deposits in the arteries

Risk factors:

Smoking

Diabetes

High blood pressure

High cholesterol

Symptoms:

Hair loss on your legs and feet

Numbness or weakness in the legs

Brittle, slow growing toenails

Shiny skin

Diagnosis:

Physical examination by your general physician and by comparing the blood pressure in your arm and your ankle

Treatment:

No specific treatment

Statins

Anti hypertensive drugs

Anti platelets

Surgery : angioplasty.

PANDEMIC FLU

Refer influenza

PARA INFLUENZA

Refer HPIV

PNEUMONIA

Definition:

Pneumonia is a serious infection caused by Streptococcus pneumonia

Epidemiology:

Worldwide

Pathophysiology:

Infects the lungs

Risk factors:

Weekend immune system

Solid organ transplant

Blood cancer

Stem cell transplant

Inflammatory diseases

Symptoms:

Fever

Cough

Hemoptysis

Difficulty in breathing

Chestpain

Fatigue

Diagnosis:

Chest X ray

PCR

Treatment:

Trimethoprim / sulfamethoxazole

POX VIRUS INFECTION

Refer chicken pox

PRION DISEASE

Prion diseases:

CJD, CWD and bovine spongiform encephalopathy.

PROSTATE CANCER

Definition:

Prostate cancer, is the development of cancer in the prostate gland in male reproductive system.

Epidemiology:

Worldwide

Pathophysiology:

Abnormal growth of cells in prostate

Risk factors:

Older age

Family history

Race

Symptoms:

May be asymptomatic

Difficulty urinating

Blood in urine

Pain in pelvis

Diagnosis:

Tissue biopsy

Medical imaging

Treatment:

Active surveillance

Surgery

Radiation therapy

Hormone therapy

Chemo therapy.

PSITTACOSIS

Definition:

It is also known as parrot fever.

Epidemiology:

Argentina

Australia

England

Pathophysiology:

Respiratory infection caused by bacterium Chlamydia psittaci

Risk factors:

Exposure to bacteria

Symptoms:

Fever

Chills

Nausea

Vomiting

Muscle and joint pain

Diarrhea

Weakness

Fatigue

Diagnosis:

Chest X ray

Treatment:

Tetracycline

Doxycycline

Azithromycin.

PULMONARY HYPERTENSION

Definition:

Pulmonary hypertension is a condition of increased blood pressure within the arteries of lungs

Epidemiology:

1000 new cases per year

Pathophysiology:

Increased blood pressure within the arteries of lung

Risk factors:

Family history

Prior blood clots

HIV

Sickle cell disease

COPD

Sleep apnea

Symptoms:

Shortness of breath

Syncope

Tiredness

Chestpain

Swelling of legs

Fast heart rate

Diagnosis:

Phonocardiogram

Echocardiography

Physical examination

Treatment:

Calcium channel blockers

Vaso active substances

Prostaglandins

Phosphodiesterase type 5 inhibitors.

PULMONARY EMBOLISM

Definition:

Pulmonary embolism is a blockage of an artery in the lungs by a substance that has moved from elsewhere in the body through blood stream.

Epidemiology:

50,000 to 2,00,000 deaths per year

Pathophysiology:

PE usually results from a blood clot in the leg that travels to the lung

Risk factors:

Cancer

Prolonged bed rest

Smoking

Stroke

Certain genetic conditions

Estrogen based medication

Pregnancy

Obesity

Symptoms:

Shortness of breath

Chest pain

Hemoptysis

Diagnosis:

CT

Lung ventilation or perfusion scan

Treatment:

Blood thinners such as heparin or warfarin.

PELVIC INFLAMMATORY DISEASE [PID]

Definition:

PID is an infection of the upper part of female reproductive system

Epidemiology:

Worldwide

Pathophysiology:

Bacteria that spread from vagina and cervix

Risk factors:

Gonorrhea

Chlamydia

Symptoms:

Fever

Cervical motion tenderness

Lower abdominal pain

New or different discharge

Uterine tenderness

Diagnosis:

Tissue biopsy

CT

MRI

ESR

CRP

Treatment:

Antibiotic therapy

Cefoxitin plus doxycycline

Clindamycin plus gentamicin.

PHTHIRIASIS

Definition:

The state or condition of being infested with lice

Epidemiology:

The prevalence of phthiriasis is unknown

Pathophysiology:

Lice infestation

Risk factors:

Sexual contact

Secondary bacterial infection can occur from scratching of the skin

Symptoms:

Itching

Live lice may also be visible to the unaided eye

Diagnosis:

Stereo-microscope

Treatment:

Lice killing lotion containing pyrethrins and piperonyl

.

PINWORM INFECTION

Definition:

Pinworm infection, also known as enterobiasis, is a human parasitic disease caused by pinworm

Epidemiology:

Worldwide

Pathophysiology:

Infection caused by pinworm

Risk factors:

Contact with people who are infected

Symptoms:

Itchy anal area

Weight loss

Irritability

Insomnia

Diagnosis:

Diagnosis is by seeing the worms or eggs under a microscope.

Treatment:

Mebendazole

Pyrantel pamoate.

PLAQUE

Definition:

Dental plaque :

A sticky film that coats teeth and contain bacteria

Epidemiology:

More than 10 million cases per year

Pathophysiology:

Plaque develops when food that contains carbohydrates, such as milk, soft drink, raisins, cakes that left on the teeth

Risk factors:

Improper dental hygiene

Symptoms:

Receding gums

Bad breath

Pain or bleeding gums

Diagnosis:

Physical examination

Treatment:

Treatment depends on severity

Regular brushing and flossing can help prevent dental plaque.

PERTUSSIS

Definition:

It is also known as whooping cough, is a highly contagious respiratory disease.

Epidemiology:

Most cases occur in the developing world.

Pathophysiology:

After the bacteria are inhaled, they initially adhere to the ciliated epithelium in the nasopharynx.

Risk factors:

Air borne

Cough and sneezes of infected person

Spread from other animals

Symptoms:

Paroxysmal cough

Fainting or vomiting after coughing

Sub conjunctival hemorrhages

Uterine incontinence

Hernias

Diagnosis:

Culture

PCR

DFA

Treatment:

Erythromycin

Clarithromycin.

PLAGUE

Definition:

Plague is an infectious disease caused by bacterium Yersinia pestis

Epidemiology:

Globally about 600 cases reported a year

Pathophysiology:

Infectious disease

Risk factors:

Droplet contact

Direct physical contact

Indirect contact

Airborne transmission

Fecal oral transmission

Vector borne transmission

Symptoms:

Fever

Weakness

Headache

Diagnosis:

Finding the bacterium in a lymphnode, blood and sputum

Treatment:

Antibiotics

Supportive care

Gentamicin and fluoroquinolone.

POLIO INFECTION

Definition:

Poliomyelitis, often called as polio or infantile paralysis is an infectious disease caused by poliovirus.

Epidemiology:

Worldwide

Pathophysiology:

Infectious disease

Risk factors:

Spread by fecal-oral route

Symptoms:

Muscle weakness resulting in an inability to move

Diagnosis:

Finding the virus in the feces or antibodies in the blood

Treatment:

Supportive care

Prevention: polio vaccine.

PONTIAC FEVER

Refer legionellosis

Q FEVER

Definition:

Coxiella burnefti is an obligate intracellular bacterial pathogen causing Qfever

Epidemiology:

Population level, incidence estimates are lacking

Pathophysiology:

Inside the hostcell, invading bacterial pathogens typically subvert phagosomal maturation using a variety of mechanism

Risk factors:

Vegetarians

Farmers

Symptoms:

Abdomen, muscle pain

Fatigue

High fever

Malaise

Chills

Night sweats

Diagnosis:

Measurement of vcbx

Doxycycline

Hydroxychloroquine.

RHEUMATOID ARTHRITIS

Definition:

Rheumatoid arthritis is an autoimmune disease that can cause jointpain and damage throughout your body

Epidemiology:

Worldwide

Oldage

Pathophysiology:

Auto immune

Risk factors:

Age above 40-50years

Family history

Symptoms:

Joint pain

Joint swelling

Joint stiffness

Loss of joint function

Diagnosis:

Physical examination

Ultrasound

Xray

MRI

Blood tests:

Rheumatoid factor test

Anti-CCP

Antinuclear antibody test

ESR

C-reactive protein

Treatment:

Medications

NSAID'S

Corticosteroids

Acetaminophen

DMARD'S

Biologics.

RABIES

Definition:

Rabies is a deadly virus that attacks the CNS.

Epidemiology:

In US, one or two people die from rabies each year

Pathophysiology:

Rabies is a viral illness spread via saliva of an infected animal

Risk factors:

Travelling in areas where rabies is more common

Symptoms:

Weakness

Fever

Headache

Anxiety or confusion

Hallucinations

Hypersalivation

Hydrophobia

Difficulty swallowing

Diagnosis:

Testing saliva, blood samples, spinal fluid and skin samples

Treatment:

No specific treatment

Series of rabies vaccine

RAT-BITE FEVER

Definition:

Rat-bite fever is an acute, febrile human illness caused by bacteria transmitted by rodents, in most cases, which is passed from rodent to human by rodent's urine or mucus secretions.

Epidemiology:

US

Europe

Australia

Africa

Most common: japan

Pathophysiology:

Bacteria pass from rodent to human

Risk factors:

Contaminated food and water

Household pets

Symptoms:

Inflammation around the open sore

Rash

Chills

Fever

Vomiting

Headache

Muscle aches

Diagnosis:

Detecting bacteria in skin, blood, joint fluid or lymph nodes

Blood antibody tests

Treatment:

Pencillin

Azithromycin

Tetracyclines.

RELAPSING FEVER

Refer louse borne relapsing fever

RESPIRATORY SYNCYTIAL VIRUS INFECTION

Definition:

Human respiratory syncytial virus [HRSV] is a syncytial virus that causes respiratory tract infections.

Epidemiology:

Tropical climates

Pathophysiology:

Infection caused by HRSV

Risk factors:

Exposure to HRSV

Symptoms:

Common cold

Minor illness

Bronchiolitis

Pneumonia

Asthma

Diagnosis:

Physical examination

Chest X ray

Skin monitoring

Blood test

Treatment:

Salbutamol

Supportive care includes fluid and oxygen.

RICKETTSIA

Definition:

It is an infection caused by intracellular bacteria

Epidemiology:

Worldwide

Pathophysiology:

Infection caused by intracellular bacteria

Risk factor:

Exposure to intracellular bacteria

Symptoms:

Fever

Headache

Muscle aches

Swollen lymph glands

Cough rash

Diagnosis:

Physical examination

Difficult to diagnose

Blood test

Skin biopsy

Treatment:

Tetracycline

Doxycycline.

RIFT VALLEY FEVER

Definition:

Rift valley fever is a viral disease that can cause mild to severe symptoms

Epidemiology:

Worldwide

Pathophysiology:

RVFV'S RNA play an important role in the virus pathology

Risk factors:

Exposure to virus

Symptoms:

Fever

Muscle aches

Head aches

Loss of sight

Infections of brain

Confusion

Liver problems

Diagnosis:

Finding antibodies or virus in the blood

Treatment:

Supportive care.

RIVER BLINDNESS

Definition:

It is also known as onchocerciasis, is a disease caused by infection with parasitic worm Onchocerca volvulus

Epidemiology:

15.5 million affected

Pathophysiology:

It is an eye and skin disease transmitted by bite of a female black fly

Risk factors:

Exposure to tick bite

Symptoms:

Itching

Bumps under the skin

Blindness

Skin atrophy

Diagnosis:

Slit lamp examination

Antibody tests

Treatment:

Anti parasitic drug: ivermectin

Doxycycline: antibiotic.

ROTA VIRUS

Definition:

Rotavirus is the most common cause of diarrheal disease among infants and young children

Epidemiology:

Nearly every child in the world is infected with rotavirus atleast once by the age of 5

Pathophysiology:

The virus is transmitted by the fecal-oral route. It infects and damages the cells that line small intestine and cause gastroenteritis

Risk factors:

Exposure to virus

Symptoms:

Nausea

Vomiting

Watery diarrhea

Low grade fever

Diagnosis:

RT-PCR

Stool examination

Treatment:

Management of dehydration

IV therapy

Probiotics.

RUBELLA

Refer German measles

RUNNY NOSE

Definition:

Rhinorrhea [runny nose] is a condition where the nasal cavity is filled with significant amount of mucus fluid.

Epidemiology:

Worldwide

Pathophysiology:

Nasal cavity is filled with significant amount of mucus fluid

Risk factos:

Cold temperature

Symptoms:

Sneezing

Sinusitis

Coughing

Nose bleeds

Nasal discharge

Diagnosis:

Physical observation

Treatment:

Mostly not necessary

Saline nasal sprays

Anti histamines.

SALMONELLA INFECTION:

Definition:

Infection caused by salmonella gram-negative, rod shaped bacilli

Epidemiology:

Affects around 1.4 million americans every year

Pathophysiology:

Infection caused by salmonella

Risk factors:

Uncooked food

Lack of hygiene

Keeping pet reptile

Symptoms:

Stomach cramps

Bloody stools

Chills

Diarrhea

Fever

Headache

Musclepains

Diagnosis:

Blood and stool tests

Treatment:

Fluid

Antibiotics

Antimotility drugs.

SAPPINIA INFECTION

Definition:

Infection caused by sappinia- free living ameba species

Epidemiology:

Worldwide

Pathophysiology:

Infection caused by sappinia

Risk factors:

Exposure to sappinia usually found in elk, buffalo feces, soil containing rotting plants

Symptoms:

Head ache

Sensitivity to light

Nausea

Stomach upset

Vomiting

Blurry vision

Loss of consciousness

Diagnosis:

Based on symptoms

Samples of CSF and brain tissue

Treatment:

Removal of tumor in the brain

Series of drugs given to patient after surgery.

SCABIES

Definition:

Scabies, also known as seven-year itch, is a contagious skin infestation by the mite Sarcoptes scabies

Epidemiology:

Worldwide

Pathophysiology:

Contagious skin infestation by the mite Sarcoptes scabies

Risk factors:

Sarcoptes scabies mite spread by close contact

Symptoms:

Itchiness

Pimple like rash

Diagnosis:

Physical examination

Treatment:

Permethrin

Lindane

Ivermectin.

SCARLET FEVER

Definition:

It is a disease which can occur as a result of group A streptococcus infection

Epidemiology:

Worldwide

Pathophysiology:

Group A streptococcus infection

Risk factors:

Unhygienic conditions

Contact with sick people

Exposure

Symptoms:

Sore throat

Fever

Head ache

Swollen lymph nodes

Characteristic rash

Tongue may be red and bumpy

Diagnosis:

Throat culture

Treatment:

Antibiotic therapy:

Pencillin V

Amoxicillin.

SCHISTOSOMA INFECTION

Definition:.

Infection caused by schistosoma

Epidemiology:

4,400 to 2,00,000 deaths

Pathophysiology:

Infection caused by schistosoma spread by contact with fresh water contaminated with parasites

Risk factors:

Contact with fresh water contaminated with parasite

Symptoms:

Abdominal pain

Diarrhea

Bloody stool

Blood in urine

Liver damage

Kidney failure

Infertility

Diagnosis:

Finding eggs of the parasite in urine or stool

Antibodies in blood

Treatment:

Praziquantel

Oxamniquine.

SEIZURES

Refer epilepsy

SEASONAL FLU

Refer influenza

SEPTISEMIA

Definition:

Septicemia is a serious blood stream infection. Sepsis is a serious complication of septicemia.

Epidemiology:

1 million every year

Pathophysiology:

Serious blood stream infection

Risk factors:

UTI

Lung infections

Kidney infections

Infections in the abdominal area

Mechanical ventilation

Symptoms:

Chills

Elevated body temperature

Very fast respiration

Rapid heart rate

Reduced urine volume

Red dots that appear on the skin

Inadequate blood flow

Diagnosis:

X ray

MRI

CT scans

Ultrasound

Treatment:

Broad spectrum antibiotics.

SPOTTED FEVER

Refer rickettsia

SHIGELLA INFECTION

Definition:

This is a type of gastroenteritis caused by shigella bacteria

Epidemiology:

Worldwide

Pathophysiology:

Inflammation of stomach and intestine

Risk factors:

Contaminated food and water

Symptoms:

Diarrhea

Fever

Vomiting

Stomach cramps

Diagnosis:

Fecal sample

PCR

Treatment:

Specific antibiotic therapy

Supportive care.

SICKLE CELL DISEASE

Definition:

SCD is a group of blood disorders typically inherited from a person's parents

Epidemiology:

Worldwide

Pathophysiology:

Round and biconcave RBC becomes sickle cell shape

Risk factors:

Genetic

Symptoms:

Attacks of pain

Anemia

Swelling in the hands and feet

Bacterial infections

Stroke

Diagnosis:

Complete blood count

Chromatography

Treatment:

Vaccination

Antibiotics

High fluid intake

Folic acid supplementation

Pain medication

Blood transfusions.

SINUS INFECTION

Definition:

It is the inflammation or swelling of the tissues lining the sinus

Epidemiology:

35 million every year

Pathophysiology:

Inflammation or swelling of tissues lining the sinus

Risk factors:

Common cold

Nasal polyps

Allergies

Smoking

Immune system disorders

Symptoms:

Facial pain

Stuffed up nose

Runny nose

Loss of smell

Cough

Congestion

Fever

Bad breath

Fatigue

Dental pain

Diagnosis:

Based on symptoms

Xray

Treatment:

Decongestant

Saline nasal washes

Antibiotics.

SKIN INFECTION

Refer impetigo

SKIN CANCER

Definition:

Skin cancer is the uncontrolled growth of cancer cells in the skin

Epidemiology:

Affecting 1 in 5 americans during their life times

Pathophysiology:

Uncontrolled growth of cancer cells in the skin

Risk factors:

Prolonged exposure to UV rays

Over the age of 40

Family history

Fair complexion

Received an organ transplant

Symptoms:

Changes in the skin that donot heal

Ulcering the skin

Discoloured skin

Changes in the existing males

Diagnosis:

Tissue biopsy

Treatment:

Surgery

Radiation therapy

Fluorouracil.

SLEEPING SICKNESS

Refer African trypanosomiasis

SMALL POX

Definition:

Small pox is an extremely contagious and deadly virus for which there is no known cure

Epidemiology:

Widespread smallpox epidemics

Pathophysiology:

Caused by virus : Variola major, Variola minor

Risk factors:

Contact with the person having small pox

Symptoms:

High fever

Chills

Headache

Severe backpain

Abdominal pain

Vomiting

Diagnosis:

Physical observation

Treatment:

No cure

Supportive therapy.

SORE THROAT

Definition:

It is a painful, dry, scratchy feeling in the throat

Epidemiology:

Worldwide

Pathophysiology:

Pharyngitis

Tonsillitis

Laryngitis

Risk factors:

Cold

Strep throat

Bacterial infections

Allergies

GERD

Tumor

Smoke

Chemicals

Symptoms:

Throat:

Scratchy

Burning

Raw

Dry

Tender

Diagnosis:

Based on symptoms

Throat culture

Treatment:

Azithromycin

Ibuprofen

Acetaminophen.

SPINA BIFIDA

Definition:

It is a birth defect where there is incomplete closing of the back bones and membranes around the spinal cord.

Epidemiology:

1 to 5 per 1000 births

Pathophysiology:

Incomplete closing of back bones and membranes around the spinal cord.

Risk factors:

Genetic

Environmental

Symptoms:

Hairy patch

Dimple

Dark spot

Swelling on the lower back

Diagnosis:

Based on symptoms

Medical imaging

Treatment:

Surgery

Physiotherapy.

SPIRILLUM MINUS INFECTION

Refer rat-bite fever

STREP INFECTION

Refer sore throat

STRESS

Stress is a feeling of strain and pressure

Stress can increase the risk of:

Stroke

Heart attack

Ulcers

Mental illness such as depression

Reduce your stress levels to lead a healthy and happy life.

Psychological counselling may be necessary.

SUDDEN INFANT DEATH SYNDROME

Definition:

SIDS is the sudden unexplained death of child less than one year of age.

Epidemiology:

1 in 1000 to 10000

Risk factors:

Sleeping on stomach

Over heating

Exposure to tobacco smoke

Bed sharing

Symptoms:

Death

Prevention:

Putting newborns on their back to sleep

Pacifier

Breast feeding

Immunization

STROKE

Definition:

It is a medical condition in which poor blood flow to the brain results in cell death.

Epidemiology:

Worldwide

Pathophysiology:

Poor blood flow to the brain

It might be due to deposition of cholesterol,etc

Risk factors:

High blood pressure

Smoking

Obesity

High blood cholesterol

Diabetes mellitus

Atrial fibrillation

Symptoms:

Inability to feel

Problems understanding or speaking

Feeling like the world is spinning

Loss of vision to one side

Diagnosis:

CT

MRI

Doppler ultrasound

Arteriography

Blood test

Treatment:

Tissue plasminogen activator

Anti platelet

Anti thrombotics

Statins.

SWINE INFLUENZA

Definition:

Swine influenza is an infection caused by any one of the several types of swine influenza viuses.

Epidemiology:

The 2009 outbreak of swineflu that infected humans was of the H1N1 subtype

Pathophysiology:

Infection caused by one of the several types of swine influenza viruses.

Risk factors:

People aged over 65years

Children under 5 years

People with chronic diseases

Pregnant women

Immune compromised individuals

Symptoms:

Body aches

Chills

Cough

Headache

Sorethroat

Fever

Tiredness

Diagnosis:

Rapid influenza diagnostic test

Treatment:

Amantadine

Rimantidine

Zanamivir and oseltamivir inhibit influenza neuraminidase protein.

SYPHILIS

Definition:

It is a sexually transmitted infection caused by bacterium Treponema pallidum

Epidemiology:

Worldwide

Pathophysiology:

Sexually transmitted infection

Risk factors:

Prostitution

Decreasing use of condoms

Unsafe sexual practices

Symptoms:

Firm, painless, non itchy skin ulcer

4stages:

Primary

Secondary

Latent

Tertiary

Congenitally

Diagnosis:

Blood tests:

Treponemal

Non-treponemal

Treatment:

IM benzathine benzyl pencillin

Doxycycline

Tetracycline

Ceftriaxone.

SYSTEMIC LUPUS ERYTHEMATOSUS

Definition:

It is an auto-immune disease

Epidemiology:

Worldwide

Pathophysiology:

Autoimmune

Risk factors:

Genetics

Environmental:

UV rays

Certain medications

Viruses

Physical or emotional stress

Trauma

Symptoms:

Severe fatigue

Joint pain

Joint swelling

Head aches

A rash on cheeks

Hairloss

Anemia

Blood clotting problems

Fingers turning white or blue

Diagnosis:

Blood tests:

Antibody tests

Complete blood count

Urine analysis

Chest X ray

Treatment:

Anti-inflammatory medications

Steroid creams for rashes

Corticosteroids

Antimalarial drugs.

TAENIA INFECTION

Definition:

It is a parasitic infection caused by tapeworm

Epidemiology:

Worldwide

Pathophysiology:

Parasitic infections caused by tapeworm

Risk factors:

Eating raw or uncooked beef

Poor sanitation

Surrounded with cattle

Poor hygiene

HIV

AIDS

Organ transplant

Diabetes

Symptoms:

Pain

Unexplained weight loss

Blockage of intestine

Digestive problems

Diagnosis:

Complete blood count

Stool examination

Treatment:

Anthelminthics

Praziquantel.

TAPEWORM INFECTION

Definition:

Infection caused by tapeworm – intestinal parasite

Epidemiology:

Worldwide

Pathophysiology:

Infection caused by tapeworm

Risk factors:

Exposure to tapeworm

Symptoms:

Abdominal pain

Vomiting

Nausea

Weight loss

Inflammation of intestine

Diarrhea

Altered appetite

Diagnosis:

Stool examination

Treatment:

Anti inflammatory drugs

Cyst surgery.

TUBERCULOSIS

Definition:

It is an infectious disease that usually affects lungs

Epidemiology:

Worldwide

Pathophysiology:

Infection to lungs caused by Mycobacterium tuberculosis which is an aerobic pathogen.

Risk factors:

Smoking

HIV

AIDS

Person to person

Symptoms:

Chronic cough

Fever

Blood in sputum

Weight loss

Diagnosis:

Patch test

Sputum test

Chest X ray

Treatment:

First line:

Rifampicin

Isoniazide

Pyremethamide

Ethambutal

Second line:

Streptomycin

Canamycin.

TRAUMATIC BRAIN INJURY

Definition:

It results from a violent blow or jolt to the head or object

Epidemiology:

World wide

Pathophysiology:

Results from a violent blow

Risk factors:

Falls

Vehicle related illness

Violence

Sports injuries

Symptoms:

Loss of consciousness

Persistent headache

Repeated vomiting or nausea

Convulsions

Seizures

Inability to awaken from sleep

Loss of coordination

Weakness or numbness in the fingers and toes

Diagnosis:

Glasgow coma scale

CT

MRI

Treatment:

Immediate emergency care

Medications:

Diuretics

Anti-seizure drugs

Coma inducing drugs

Surgery.

TESTICULAR CANCER

Definition:

Testicular cancer occurs in the testicles, which are located inside the scrotum, a loose bag of skin underneath the penis

Epidemiology:

Worldwide

Age: 15 to 35

Male

Pathophysiology:

Abnormal growth of cancer cells

Risk factors:

An undescended testicle

Abnormal testicle development

Family history

Symptoms:

A lump or enlargement in either testicle

A feeling of heaviness in the scrotum

A dull ache in the abdomen and groin

A sudden collection of fluid in the scrotum

Pain or discomfort in a testicle

Back pain

Diagnosis:

Self examination to check lumps

Ultrasound

Bloodtests

Treatment:

Surgery

Radiation therapy

Chemotherapy.

TETANUS INFECTION

Definition:

Tetanus, also known as lock jaw, is an infection characterized by muscle spasms.

Epidemiology:

Worldwide

Pathophysiology:

Begin in the jaw caused by Clostridium tetani

Risk factors:

Break in the skin

Exposure to clostridium tetani

Symptoms:

Muscle spasms

Fever

Headache

Diagnosis:

Based on symptoms

Treatment:

Tetanus immune globulin

Muscle relaxants

Mechanical ventilation.

THALASSEMIA

Definition:

Thalassemia are inherited blood disorders characterized by abnormal hemoglobin production.

Epidemiology:

Worldwide

Pathophysiology:

Abnormal hemoglobin production

Risk factors:

Genetic disorders

Inherited

Symptoms:

Feeling tired

Pale skin

Enlarged spleen

Yellowish skin

Dark urine

Diagnosis:

Blood tests

Genetic tests

Treatment:

Blood transfusions

Iron chelation

Folic acid.

THORACIC AORTIC ANEURYSM

Definition:

A thoracic aortic aneurysm is a weekend area in the upper part of aorta

Epidemiology:

Worldwide

Pathophysiology:

Weekend area in the upper part of aorta

Risk factors:

Atherosclerosis

Genetic conditions

Untreated infections

Traumatic injury

Symptoms:

Tenderness or pain in the chest

Back pain

Hoarseness

Cough

Shortness of breath

Diagnosis:

Chest X ray

CT

MRI

Ultrasound

Treatment:

Surgery

Beta blockers

ARB'S

Statins.

THROMBOPHILIA

Definition:

Thrombophilia means that blood has increased tendency to form clots

Epidemiology:

Worldwide

Pathophysiology:

Blood has increased tendency to form clots

Risk factors:

Genetic

Symptoms:

Deep vein thrombosis

Pulmonary embolism

Shortness of breath

Chest pain

Palpitations

Protein deficiency

Diagnosis:

Complete blood count

Treatment:

Anti coagulation medications.

THROMBOSIS

It is an abnormality of blood coagulation that results the risk of thrombophilia

Refer thrombophilia

TINEA

Refer skin infection

TOURETTE SYNDROME

Definition:

It is a neuropsychiatric disorder with onset in childhood

Epidemiology:

About 1%

Pathophysiology:

Neuropsychiatric

Risk factors:

Genetic with environmental influence

Symptoms:

Repeatedly blinking of eyes

Shrugging shoulders

Offensive words

Diagnosis:

Based on history and symptoms

Treatment:

Education

Behavioral therapy

Antipsychotics.

TOXOCARA INFECTION

Definition:

It is an infection transmitted from animals to humans

Epidemiology:

Worldwide

Pathophysiology:

Infection

Risk factors:

Swallowing dirt

Contaminated food and water

Symptoms:

Ocular:

Vision loss

Eye inflammation

Damage to retina

Visceral:

Fever

Fatigue

Coughing

Wheezing

Abdominal pain

Diagnosis:

Based on symptoms

Treatment:

Antiparasitic drugs.

TOXOPLASMA INFECTION

Definition:

It is an infection caused by Toxoplasma gondii

Epidemiology:

Worldwide

Pathophysiology:

Infection

Risk factors:

Exposure to infected cat feces

Symptoms:

Often none

Birth defects during pregnancy

Diagnosis:

Blood test

Amniotic fluid test

Treatment:

During pregnancy: spiramycin

Pyrimethamine

Sulfadiazene.

TYPHOID FEVER

Definition:

Bacterial infection caused by Salmonella typhi

Epidemiology:

Worldwide

Pathophysiology:

Infection

Risk factors:

Contaminated food and water

Poor sanitation

Poor hygiene

Symptoms:

Fever

Abdominal pain

Headache

Rash

Diagnosis:

Bacterial culture

Widal test

DNA detection

Treatment:

Fluoroquinolone

Ceftriaxone

Ampicillin

Chloramphenicol

Amoxicillin

Trimethoprim-sulfamethoxazole.

TRICHOMONAS INFECTION

Definition:

It is a sexually transmitted disease

Epidemiology:

Worldwide

Common

Pathophysiology:

Sexually transmitted

Risk factors:

Multiple sex partners

Sex without condom

Symptoms:

Vaginal discharge

Vaginal spotting or bleeding

Genital burning

Genital redness

Diagnosis:

Cell cultures

Antigen tests

Examining samples of vaginal fluid

Treatment:

Metronidazole

Tinidazole.

TRICHURIASIS

Definition:

Also known as whip worm infection

Epidemiology:

World wide

Pathophysiology:

Infection caused by parasitic worm

Risk factors:

Contaminated food

Symptoms:

Abdominal pain

Tiredness

Diarrhea

Diagnosis:

Stool examination

Treatment:

Albendazole

Mebendazole.

UNDULENT FEVER

Refer Brucella infection

UNEXPLAINED RESPIRATORY DISEASE OUTBREAK

Disease outbreaks are a common public health problem and investigating them can be challenging because many pathogens can cause them.

Implementing appropriate measures depend on finding a cause.

UTERINE CANCER

Definition:

Cancer of the uterus

Epidemiology:

Worldwide

Pathophysiology:

Abnormal growth of cancer cells in the uterus

Risk factors:

Being obese

High blood sugar

High blood pressure

High levels of triglycerides

Beginning menstruation at an early age

Having PCOS

Reaching menopause

Symptoms:

Vaginal bleeding

Painful urination

Pain in pelvic area

Pain during intercourse

Diagnosis:

Endometrial biopsy

Dilatation

Hysteroscopy

Xray

PET

Treatment:

Radiation therapy

Chemotherapy

Hormone therapy

Targeted therapy.

VAGINAL CANCER AND VULVAR CANCER

Definition:

Vulvar cancer affects the external genital organs of a women

Epidemiology:

Worldwide

Pathophysiology:

Abnormal growth of cancer cells

Risk factors:

Age over 70 years

HPV

Melanoma

STI'S

Smoking

Kidney transplant

HIV

Symptoms:

Painful sexual intercourse

Bleeding

Pain and burning

Painful urination

Persistent itching

Ulceration

Diagnosis:

Cystoscopy

MRI

CT

Treatment:

Laser therapy

Excision.

VALLY FEVER

Refer coccidioidomycosis

VARICELLA DISEASE

Refer chickenpox

VIRAL HEMORRHAGIC FEVER

Definition:

Viral hemorrhagic fevers are infectious diseases that interfere with the blood's ability to clot.

Epidemiology:

Worldwide

Pathophysiology:

Infectious disease

Interfere with the blood's ability to clot

Risk factors:

Working with the sick

Slaughtering infected animals

Sharing needles

Having unprotected sex

Symptoms:

High fever

Fatigue

Dizziness

Muscle, bone, joint aches

Weakness

Diagnosis:

Based on symptoms

Blood test

Treatment:

Ribavirin.

VIRAL HEPATITIS

Refer hepatitis

VIRAL MENINGITIS

Refer aseptic meningitis

VISION IMPAIRMENT

Definition:

Visual impairment, also known as vision impairment or vision loss, is a decreased ability to see to a degree that causes problems not fixable by usual means, such as glasses.

Epidemiology:

13% of population

Pathophysiology:

Vision loss

Optic nerve damage

Risk factors:

Uncorrected refractive errors

Cataracts

Glaucoma

Symptoms:

Decreased ability to see

Diagnosis:

Eye examination

Treatment:

Vision rehabilitation

Changes in the environment

Assistive devices.

VON WILLEBRAND DISEASE

Definition:

It is a life long bleeding disorder in which your blood doesn't clot well.

Epidemiology:

Worldwide

Pathophysiology:

Blood doesn't clot well

Risk factors:

Inherited from parent : faulty gene

Symptoms:

Excessive bleeding from an injury

Heavy or long menstrual bleeding

Blood in your urine or stool

Easy bruising

Diagnosis:

Von willebrand factor antigen

Factor 8 clotting activity

Treatment:

Life long condition – no cure

Desmopressin

Replacement therapies

Contraceptives.

WEST NILE VIRUS INFECTION

Definition:

West nile virus infection – is a virus infection typically spread by mosquitoes.

Epidemiology:

Worldwide

Pathophysiology:

Viral infection spread by mosquitoes

Risk factors:

Kidney conditions

Diabetes

Hypertension

Cancer

Impaired immune system

Symptoms:

Fever

Headache

Bodyaches

Nausea

Vomiting

Swollen lymph nodes

Rash on your chest, stomach or back

Diagnosis:

Simple blood test

Treatment:

Polyclonal immunoglobulin IV

WNV recombinant humanized monoclonal antibody

Corticosteroids.

WHIPWORM INFECTION

Refer trichuriasis

WHITMORE'S DISEASE

Refer Burkholderia psuedomallei infection

XENOTROPIC MURINE LUKEMIA VIRUS

XMRV is a gamma retrovirus that has been associated with chronic fatigue syndrome and prostate cancer

XMRV refers to a recently discovered retrovirus. It was first identified in 2006 in samples from men with prostate cancer

XMRV is closely related to a group of retroviruses called murine leukemia viruses which are known to cause cancer in certain mice.

YEAST INFECTION

Refer candida infection

YELLOW FEVER

Definition:

Yellow fever is a hemorrhagic condition

Epidemiology:

Worldwide

Pathophysiology:

Hemorrhagic condition

Caused by flavivirus

Transmitted by mosquitoes

Risk factors:

Exposure to mosquitoes

Symptoms:

Aching muscles

High fever

Dizziness

Headache

Loss of appetite

Nausea

Shiver

Vomiting

Diagnosis:

Blood test

ELISA

PCR

Treatment:

There is no effective antiviral medication to treat yellow fever

So treatment consists of supportive care.

YERSINIOSIS

Refer plague

ZIKA VIRUS INFECTION

Zikavirus is a virus related to dengue, westnile and other viruses.

The virus is transmitted to most people by mosquito vector

Refer dengue fever and west nile infection.

ZYCOMYCOSIS

Also known as mucormycosis

Definition:

Mucormycosis is any fungal infection caused by fungi

Epidemiology:

Very rare

Pathophysiology:

Infection caused by fungi

Risk factors:

HIV

AIDS

Uncontrolled diabetes mellitus

Lymphomas

Kidney failure

Organ transplant

Cirrhosis

Malnutrition

Symptoms:

Mucormycosis frequently infects:

Sinuses

Brain

Lungs

One sided headache

Nasal discharge [black]

Eyes swelling

Breathing difficulty

Diagnosis:

Biopsy

Treatment:

Amphotericin B immediately administered

Surgical removal of fungus ball

Isavuconazole was recently FDA approved to treat mucormycosis.